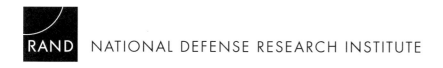

NATIONAL DEFENSE RESEARCH INSTITUTE

T0146377

Evaluation of the Operational Stress Control and Readiness (OSCAR) Program

Christine Anne Vaughan, Carrie M. Farmer, Joshua Breslau, Crystal Burnette

Prepared for the Office of the Secretary of Defense

Approved for public release; distribution unlimited

For more information on this publication, visit www.rand.org/t/RR562

Library of Congress Cataloging-in-Publication Data is available for this publication.

ISBN: 978-0-8330-9016-4

Published by the RAND Corporation, Santa Monica, Calif.

© Copyright 2015 RAND Corporation

RAND® is a registered trademark.

Limited Print and Electronic Distribution Rights

This document and trademark(s) contained herein are protected by law. This representation of RAND intellectual property is provided for noncommercial use only. Unauthorized posting of this publication online is prohibited. Permission is given to duplicate this document for personal use only, as long as it is unaltered and complete. Permission is required from RAND to reproduce, or reuse in another form, any of its research documents for commercial use. For information on reprint and linking permissions, please visit www.rand.org/pubs/permissions.html.

The RAND Corporation is a research organization that develops solutions to public policy challenges to help make communities throughout the world safer and more secure, healthier and more prosperous. RAND is nonprofit, nonpartisan, and committed to the public interest.

RAND's publications do not necessarily reflect the opinions of its research clients and sponsors.

Support RAND

Make a tax-deductible charitable contribution at
www.rand.org/giving/contribute

www.rand.org

Preface

In the past several years, the U.S. Department of Defense (DoD) has implemented numerous programs to assist U.S. military service members and their family members in coping with stressors associated with multiple and extended deployments and exposure to combat. To understand the impact of these programs on service members and their families, the Defense Centers of Excellence for Psychological Health and Traumatic Brain Injury (DCoE) asked the RAND Corporation to catalog (Weinick et al., 2011) and evaluate DoD-sponsored programs addressing psychological health. One of the programs selected for evaluation was the Marine Corps Operational Stress Control and Readiness (OSCAR) program.

The OSCAR program is designed to enhance the prevention, identification, and treatment of combat and operational stress problems among Marines by (1) embedding mental health professionals at the regiment level and (2) increasing the combat and operational stress–control capabilities of select medical, religious ministry, and operational leadership personnel. Toward this goal, select officers and noncommissioned officers attend a course that provides instruction in the principles of combat and operational stress control as practiced in the Navy and Marine Corps and training in the appropriate recognition, intervention, and referral of Marines with potential mental health problems.

Our evaluation of the OSCAR program had four main components: (1) longitudinal pre- and postdeployment surveys of Marines from OSCAR-trained and non–OSCAR-trained battalions, (2) longitudinal pre- and postdeployment surveys of OSCAR team members, (3) focus groups with Marines, and (4) semistructured interviews with commanding officers of battalions that had received OSCAR training. This report describes the findings and recommendations from this evaluation, shedding light on OSCAR's impact on the climate of stress response and recovery within the Marine Corps, as well as perceptions of OSCAR and its impact on this climate among lower-ranking Marines, small-unit leaders, and commanding officers.

The results of this report will be of particular interest to Marine Corps leadership, Headquarters Marine Corps personnel who oversee the administration and implementation of OSCAR, and national policymakers within DoD working to ensure the mental health of service members. Researchers working to understand the effects of military psychological health programs on stress-related attitudes and behaviors and mental health of military service members will also be interested in these findings.

This research was sponsored by DCoE and conducted within the Forces and Resources Policy Center of the RAND National Defense Research Institute, a federally funded research and development center sponsored by the Office of the Secretary of Defense, the Joint Staff, the Unified Combatant Commands, the Navy, the Marine Corps, the defense agencies, and the defense Intelligence Community. For more information on the RAND Forces and Resources

Policy Center, see http://www.rand.org/nsrd/ndri/centers/frp.html or contact the director (contact information is provided on the web page).

Contents

Figures and Tables

Figures

Tables

Summary

Combat and military operations expose Marines, as they do all U.S. military service members, to extremes of psychological stress. In response to the 1999 U.S. Department of Defense (DoD) Directive 6490.5 on combat stress–control programs, Marine Corps leadership designed an innovative in-unit stress-mitigation program, Operational Stress Control and Readiness (OSCAR). The OSCAR program is designed to enhance the prevention, identification, and treatment of combat and operational stress problems by integrating psychiatric expertise, concepts, and tools—traditionally the domain of medical and psychiatric professionals—into military culture. OSCAR is innovative in that it complements the Marine Corps tradition of small-unit leadership by training select Marine Corps leaders to identify and assist Marines affected by combat-related stress.

This report describes findings from an evaluation of the OSCAR program's success in achieving its key objectives of improving the prevention, identification, and management of combat and operational stress problems among Marines and, in turn, decreasing their mental health problems. We focus on the performance of OSCAR as it pertains to Marines' experiences with its implementation in Iraq and Afghanistan, conflicts recognized for high exposure to combat, as well as multiple, extended deployments.

The OSCAR evaluation had two primary aims: (1) to determine the impact of OSCAR on such outcomes as stress-related attitudes, help-seeking for stress problems, and mental health and alcohol use problems, and (2) to determine Marine Corps leaders' perceptions of OSCAR's impact on attitudes toward stress response and recovery; unit cohesion and morale; stigma around mental health and help-seeking; and unit leaders' abilities to prevent, identify, and manage stress problems in the unit. To this end, the OSCAR evaluation consisted of four components: (1) longitudinal pre- and postdeployment surveys of Marines from OSCAR-trained and non–OSCAR-trained battalions, i.e., the individual Marine survey, (2) longitudinal pre- and postdeployment surveys of OSCAR team members, i.e., the team member survey, (3) focus groups with Marines, and (4) semistructured interviews with commanding officers of battalions that had received OSCAR training. The remainder of this summary describes the key findings, conclusions, and recommendations from this evaluation.

Overview of OSCAR

The OSCAR program was originally conceived of as a new partnership between psychiatry and the military. In the early years of the program, mental health professionals were embedded at the regiment level, but, over time, OSCAR has evolved to extend mental health resources down to the battalion and company levels through the deployment of *OSCAR teams*. The OSCAR teams are made up of embedded mental health care professionals (OSCAR providers), selected medical and religious ministry personnel (OSCAR extenders), and selected officers and noncommissioned officers (NCOs) (OSCAR team members). All OSCAR program personnel receive training in combat and operational stress–control principles and management practices prior to a combat deployment. The cornerstones of OSCAR's approach to combat and operational stress control are the Combat and Operational Stress Continuum, a tool for identifying combat stress problems of varying severity, and Combat and Operational Stress First Aid (COSFA), a psychological first aid intervention for combat and operational stress.

The OSCAR program was designed to work through the actions of people trained to identify combat stress problems and react quickly and appropriately. The program was also designed to have a broad cultural impact by reducing the stigma attached to combat stress reactions and mental health care. In so doing, OSCAR is expected to have a positive effect on long-term outcomes of interest, including better mental health, lower levels of alcohol use, and lower levels of functional impairment. Figure S.1 depicts a logic model summarizing the program's desired outcomes from OSCAR personnel training (predeployment) to long-term goals (distal goals).

Figure S.1
OSCAR Logic Model

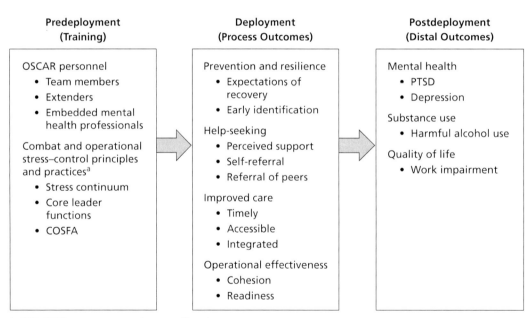

NOTE: PTSD = posttraumatic stress disorder.
[a] Combat and operational stress–control principles and practices are presented in OSCAR training but are not unique to OSCAR. Rather, they are broadly endorsed by both the Marine Corps and Navy and are presented to Marines in multiple venues.
RAND *RR562-S.1*

Individual Marine Survey

A quasi-experimental study was conducted to examine OSCAR's impact on a wide array of short- and long-term outcomes. A sample of 1,307 Marines in units deploying to Afghanistan or Iraq sometime between March 2010 and December 2011 were surveyed before and after deployment to assess stress-related attitudes, behaviors, and psychological and behavioral health. The study compared Marines in battalions that had received OSCAR training prior to deployment (i.e., OSCAR-trained battalions) with Marines in battalions that had not received OSCAR training (i.e., non–OSCAR-trained battalions) to determine whether Marines in the OSCAR-trained battalions had fared better from pre- to postdeployment on the outcomes assessed in the survey than the Marines in the non–OSCAR-trained battalions. The quasi-experimental design meant that the assignment of Marines to OSCAR-trained and non–OSCAR-trained battalions was not random. Thus, all comparisons were made with statistical adjustment, i.e., propensity score adjustment and covariate adjustment, for differences between Marines in OSCAR-trained and non–OSCAR-trained battalions in baseline characteristics and deployment experiences that could potentially confound OSCAR's effects on outcomes. Data collection began in March 2010 and concluded in October 2012.

OSCAR Increases the Use of Support for Stress Problems, but There Was No Evidence of an Impact on Marines' Mental Health Status or Any Other Outcomes

The survey results suggest that OSCAR had its intended effect on some of the proximal outcomes but did not have an impact on the distal outcomes. In particular, Marines in the OSCAR-trained battalions were more likely than Marines in the control battalions to report that they sought help for their own stress problems from fellow Marines, leaders, and corpsmen. At the same time, OSCAR did not appear to affect help-seeking from formal medical sources of care. This pattern of results persisted after statistical adjustment for traumatic experiences during deployment and participants' reactions to their most stressful deployment-related experiences.

We did not find evidence that OSCAR had its intended effect on the more-distal outcomes assessed in the survey, including probable major depression, probable PTSD, current stress levels, alcohol use, and such attitudes as expectations for stress response and recovery and stigmatization of help-seeking behavior. In fact, for some mental health measures, outcomes were worse in the OSCAR-trained battalions than in the control battalions, although these differences did not reach statistical significance when the level of exposure to traumatic events and other deployment-related stressors were taken into account.

The survey findings should be interpreted in light of the fact that all of the control battalions were combat service support, while the OSCAR-trained battalions were mostly infantry. This means that members of the OSCAR-trained battalions were likely to have had more-stressful experiences during combat than members of the control battalions. We assessed exposure and response to deployment-related stressors, but it is possible that these assessments did not capture the full extent of variation between these groups in their deployment experiences. Greater exposure to stressors might have accounted for the observed increase in help-seeking among the OSCAR-trained battalions. However, it is notable that the same pattern was not observed for help-seeking from formal clinical sources, which presumably would have been affected by the same factors.

The survey findings should also be interpreted in light of the fact that Marines in both the OSCAR-trained and control battalions reported high levels of stress-related trainings in the T1 (predeployment) survey. Specifically, 84 percent of Marines in the OSCAR-trained group and 97 percent of Marines in the control group reported one or more prior stress-related trainings, and more than 60 percent of the control group had received four or more stress-related trainings. Thus, the comparison between Marines in the OSCAR-trained and control battalions, which is the primary focus of this evaluation component, reflects the incremental contribution of OSCAR over and above the stress-related training that all Marines receive.

We also examined variation in outcomes by battalion among only the OSCAR-trained battalions. We found significant differences across the OSCAR-trained battalions in changes over time on all of the outcomes examined, providing support for the hypothesis that the implementation of OSCAR might have varied among battalions. We note, however, that there might be other reasons that outcomes varied across battalions.

Team Member Survey

The OSCAR team member survey was designed to assess OSCAR team members' perceptions of the impact of OSCAR before and after deployment. Participants in the team member survey were officers and NCOs from the same six OSCAR-trained battalions that completed the individual Marine survey; 206 OSCAR team members completed the predeployment survey, and 91 OSCAR team members completed the postdeployment survey.

Predeployment Expectations and Postdeployment Perceptions of OSCAR's Impact Were Generally Positive or Neutral

In general, prior to deployment, survey participants reported positive expectations of OSCAR's ability to positively influence unit cohesion, mission readiness, and morale and of leadership's ability to manage combat and operational stress problems in their units. However, the postdeployment surveys revealed that most team members believed that, in practice, OSCAR had less effect on these domains than they had initially expected. The survey results also suggested that team members only infrequently received requests for assistance with stress-related problems, either before or after deployment. This could explain in part why team members' perceptions of the OSCAR program's impact after deployment were lower than their expectations of OSCAR before deployment—because OSCAR team members might have been disappointed at having little opportunity during deployment to apply the principles and practices learned in OSCAR training. OSCAR team members were also asked whether, if it were up to them, the OSCAR budget would be eliminated, decreased, increased, or kept the same. Despite team members' muted expectations about the effectiveness of the program, the majority of respondents indicated that they would increase the budget for OSCAR or have it stay the same.

Focus Groups with Marines

We conducted focus groups to understand the ways in which OSCAR affects Marine Corps culture. A RAND researcher led the discussions with a set of questions developed to stimulate broad discussion of combat-related stressors, as well as more-detailed discussion about OSCAR. Participants were also asked to provide recommendations for improving the management of combat stress–related problems in the Marine Corps. Seven focus groups were sampled from five battalions; participants in the focus groups included OSCAR-trained team members, as well as NCOs and enlisted Marines, who were the intended beneficiaries of the OSCAR program but whose experience with and knowledge of the OSCAR program varied greatly.

Participants Voiced Varied Views of Combat Stress–Management Programs

Marines participating in the focus groups uniformly agreed that combat stress is a problem but emphasized that combat stress management has always been an important part of Marine Corps culture. Participants perceived OSCAR to be a set of formal methods for accomplishing goals that have always been accomplished informally. Participants frequently did not distinguish OSCAR from other combat stress–related programs, including more-general non–combat-related training on such topics as sexual harassment, and perceived that the volume of combat stress–control training Marines received is excessive. Overall, focus group members expressed a preference for nonclinical peer-to-peer approaches to combat stress and emphasized the importance of peer relations and effective leadership in combat stress management. Participants suggested that the stigma associated with mental health problems might prevent some Marines from seeking formal help, but they expressed too that an overemphasis on stress response could lead to overdiagnosis and dependence on formal care, compromising force readiness.

Participants Who Had Received OSCAR Training Appreciate It as a Platform

Participants with direct experience of the OSCAR program appreciated the value of OSCAR as a way to respond to serious combat-related stress problems without disrupting military routine. Some emphasized the ways in which the program complemented existing informal support networks. Participants also described how OSCAR is beneficial in that it provides a "common language" or "platform" for managing combat stress. Some participants stated a strong preference for OSCAR trainers with combat experience.

Interviews with Commanding Officers

Battalion commanders observe a broad range of reactions to combat among their Marines and thus can offer a valuable perspective on the management of combat-related stress and the effectiveness of the OSCAR program. We conducted 18 semistructured interviews by telephone with commanding officers of battalions that had received OSCAR training. We asked them about their views of combat stress in general, their understanding of how OSCAR addresses their needs, and their recommendations for the future.

Commanders Emphasized the Importance of Effective Leadership in Combat and Operational Stress Management

The commander interviews were remarkable for their unanimity with respect to one dominant theme: that combat and operational stress management should be viewed primarily as a problem of effective leadership rather than medical intervention. According to this view, effective leaders create cohesion and high morale in the units they lead, and cohesive units are naturally conducive to responding to stress. These responses include the early identification of behavioral change, the absence of stigma related to care-seeking, and the presence of strong peer support that can reduce the need for removing affected people for medical care. This view echoes Marines' preference for informal peer-to-peer stress support rather than formal mental health intervention.

Commanders View OSCAR as Consistent with Effective Leadership

Overwhelmingly, commanders voiced positive opinions of OSCAR because they view it as consistent with their existing principles of effective leadership. They noted how OSCAR normalizes open communication about stressful experiences and psychological reactions, provides a common language for communicating about stress, and mobilizes and reinforces peer support without involvement of external resources or authorities.

Commanders' Views of OSCAR Personnel and Training

Commanders suggested that training should not be limited to select NCOs and officers but, instead, opened to lower-ranking Marines. They also expressed the value of an OSCAR trainer with extensive combat experience or who had been seriously wounded but had gone on to have a successful Marine Corps career. There was some concern that OSCAR training would be difficult to maintain during peacetime because there would be less emphasis on combat stress in general.

Conclusions and Recommendations

Although findings from the team member survey, focus groups, and interviews collectively suggest that Marines, both enlisted and officers, widely perceive OSCAR as a useful tool for combat and operational stress control, findings from the individual Marine survey indicate that OSCAR has not fulfilled its mission of improving many of the key outcomes that it was designed to affect. Specifically, the individual Marine survey found no evidence that OSCAR significantly influenced stress-related attitudes or health-related outcomes. The lack of significant effects of OSCAR on these outcomes might be attributable to methodological limitations of the individual Marine survey—namely, limited precision to detect significant effects because of multiple statistical adjustments for confounds; variability in the implementation of OSCAR across battalions, which was suggested by findings of variability in outcomes across battalions in the OSCAR group; and the possibility that OSCAR, even if implemented consistently and with fidelity to the program's design, does not improve stress-related attitudes, help-seeking behavior, and mental health outcomes relative to the other types of stress-control training received by all Marines, including those in the non–OSCAR-trained (control) battalions.

The individual Marine survey also demonstrated that OSCAR significantly increased the use of unit resources, such as fellow Marines, leaders, and corpsmen, for stress-related problems. However, given the possibility of residual confounding of battalion type with receipt of OSCAR training, these effects might alternatively reflect a greater need for help in the OSCAR-trained battalions, which were nearly all infantry and had greater combat exposure, than the control battalions, which were all combat service support.

Thus, this evaluation did not find evidence of OSCAR's effectiveness that would support the continuation of OSCAR in its current form. In recommending a way forward for the Marine Corps in its efforts to manage combat and operational stress, we rely on findings from this evaluation's qualitative components, other research, and best practices for program improvement and implementation. Because none of the recommendations has been formally tested, we do not know the extent to which their adoption will positively affect combat and operational stress management in the Marine Corps. Moreover, some of the recommendations might be very difficult to implement in light of organizational, policy, regulatory, and budgetary constraints. Thus, the recommendations offered here should be viewed as suggestive rather than prescriptive.

Review and Streamline Marine Corps Combat and Operational Stress–Control Training Programs

The evaluation results highlighted the excess of combat and operational stress–control training received by Marines, suggesting the need for a more streamlined approach to this type of training. In integrating and streamlining combat and operational stress–control training programs, the Marine Corps might wish to consider retaining or strengthening the positive features of OSCAR and redesigning or eliminating features that were less positively perceived.

- **Identify and reduce duplication of effort in combat and operational stress–control trainings.** Marines reported receiving multiple trainings related to management of combat and operational stress, in addition to OSCAR. We recommend a thorough review of the concepts and methods of combat and operational stress–control training programs that would align the content and rationalize the scheduling of training in this area across the Marine Corps.
- **Enhance the use of a common language for concepts related to combat and operational stress control across combat and operational stress–control programs.** Findings from the qualitative components of the evaluation indicated that OSCAR was valued because of its being a shared language for talking about and managing combat and operational stress. Thus, we also recommend that, in the process of reviewing and streamlining combat and operational stress–control training, decisionmakers pay attention to consistency in the concepts and specific language across training programs and the procedures that are taught.
- **Ensure that combat and operational stress–control program trainers have combat experience.** Marines emphasized that they prefer OSCAR trainers who have combat experience. Consistent with the current OSCAR training guidelines, we recommend maintaining a pool of certified trainers who have personal experience with combat and skill in communicating the importance of combat and operational stress control to Marines.

Identify Potential Changes to the Design and Implementation of Combat and Operational Stress–Control Training

Ideas about potential changes to the design and implementation of combat and operational stress–control training that might increase the effectiveness of such training can come from many sources, including program participants, implementation literature, and other programs. Here we suggest potential changes to this training based on the findings from this evaluation:

- **Consider providing combat and operational stress–control training to all Marines in the chain of command, down to the level of squad leader.** Although some commanders value the OSCAR team members as resources for Marines experiencing combat-related stress, a consistent concern was that Marines are not likely to seek out help from someone simply because that person has been designated as a mentor. Further, the survey results show that the number of Marines seeking advice about combat stress issues from team members did not change as a result of OSCAR training. In light of these findings, we recommend that combat and operational stress–control training be provided to a broader range of people in leadership positions so that individual consultations are not stigmatized and the effectiveness of response to combat-related stress will not be compromised.

- **Integrate combat and operational stress–control training into the deployment cycle and maintain it regularly among nondeploying troops.** Participants made two important suggestions regarding the timing of training. First, some suggested improvement to the linkage of the training to the deployment cycle, including, for instance, booster sessions and postdeployment sessions. Second, some suggested that the training be reinforced routinely, regardless of the deployment schedule—e.g., on an annual basis—in order to maintain readiness during peacetime.

Pilot Test Changes to Combat and Operational Stress–Control Training

Consistent with best practices for program development and implementation (Ryan et al., 2014), changes to the combat and operational stress–control training program should be pilot-tested on a small scale to determine its feasibility and effectiveness with respect to its impact on key outcomes. If results of the pilot test are promising, the program's implementation can be gradually expanded and assessed to identify and correct challenges of implementation that inevitably accompany program expansion.

If the pilot test is not successful, then the Marine Corps might wish to revise the program based on process improvement data collected during the pilot test and test the revised version. Alternatively, the Marine Corps might prefer to abandon this approach to stress-control training and consider shifting its investments in psychological health to other policies and programs that have a stronger evidence base.

Expand the Evidence Base Regarding Operational Stress Management

Much work remains to be done in order to learn the lessons from the initial implementation of OSCAR and use those lessons to improve combat and operational stress management in the Marine Corps. To continue improving Marine Corps methods for managing combat and operational stress, further research will be necessary. We therefore make the following recommendation:

- **Examine patterns of support-seeking and help-seeking in more detail.** Although the survey results demonstrate an increase in certain types of help-seeking in OSCAR-trained battalions, we did not study the nature of this help-seeking and the providers' response to it. Information on the process for seeking support from informal sources and help from formal sources is critical to the continuing improvement of combat and operational stress–control systems.

Acknowledgments

We gratefully acknowledge the support of our current and previous project monitors, Capt. John Golden, Yoni Tyberg, and Col. Christopher Robinson, and current and former staff at the Defense Centers of Excellence for Psychological Health and Traumatic Brain Injury, particularly CPT Dayami Liebenguth. We also acknowledge the support of our points of contact in the Marine Corps Combat and Operational Stress Control office, Patricia Powell and MSgt Michael O'Brien. We appreciate the comments provided by our reviewers, Terry Schell and William Nash. We addressed their constructive critiques, as part of RAND's rigorous quality assurance process, to improve the quality of this report. We acknowledge the support and assistance of Claude Setodji, Kate Giglio, Reema Singh, Alexandra Smith, and Anna Smith in the preparation of this report. We are also grateful to the Marines who participated in this evaluation for their time and to our points of contact at each base for their time and support.

Abbreviations

AUDIT-C	Alcohol Use Disorders Identification Test–Consumption
CI	confidence interval
CO	commanding officer
COSC	Combat and Operational Stress Control
COSFA	Combat and Operational Stress First Aid
DCoE	Defense Centers of Excellence for Psychological Health and Traumatic Brain Injury
DoD	Department of Defense
DRRI	Deployment Risk and Resilience Inventory
EAS	end of active service
HPQ	Health Performance Questionnaire
HQMC	Headquarters Marine Corps
HSPC	human subject–protection committee
IOM	Institute of Medicine
LEC	Life Events Checklist
LL	lower limit
M	mean
MARADMIN	Marine Administrative Message
MDD	major depressive disorder
MEF	Marine Expeditionary Force
NCO	noncommissioned officer
OR	odds ratio
OSCAR	Operational Stress Control and Readiness
PBQ-SR	Peritraumatic Behavior Questionnaire, Self-Rated version

PCL-C	Posttraumatic Symptom Checklist–Civilian version
PCS	permanent change of station
PDHA	Postdeployment Health Assessment
PFC	private first class
PHQ	Patient Health Questionnaire
POC	point of contact
PTSD	posttraumatic stress disorder
RP	religious program specialist
SD	standard deviation
SE	standard error
SF	Short-Form Health Survey
SgtMaj	sergeant major
T1	Time 1: predeployment OSCAR training
T2	Time 2: postdeployment OSCAR training
UL	upper limit
USMC	U.S. Marine Corps
XO	executive officer

CHAPTER ONE

Introduction

The wars in Afghanistan and Iraq have posed some challenges for U.S. military service members and their families. Among these are multiple and extended deployments and exposure to combat stressors. Although most military personnel and their families cope well with these stressors, many also experience difficulties handling stress at some point. In the past several years, the U.S. Department of Defense (DoD) has implemented numerous programs to address these issues by building resilience, preventing stress-related problems, and identifying and treating problems quickly when they occur. To understand the impact of these programs on service members and their families, the RAND Corporation has been engaged to catalog (Weinick et al., 2011) and evaluate DoD-sponsored programs addressing psychological health.

One of the programs selected for evaluation is Operational Stress Control and Readiness (OSCAR), a Marine Corps program designed to enhance the prevention, identification, and treatment of combat and operational stress problems among Marines by (1) embedding mental health professionals at the regimental level and (2) increasing the combat and operational stress–control capabilities of select medical, religious ministry, and operational leadership personnel. To achieve the latter goal, OSCAR provides predeployment training conducted at the battalion level for selected officers and noncommissioned officers (NCOs) in the prevention, identification, and treatment of combat and operational stress problems. These personnel—OSCAR mental health professionals, medical and religious ministry personnel, and select officers and NCOs—constitute the unit's OSCAR team and are expected to be able to prevent, identify, and manage stress problems within the unit. The OSCAR team enhances the ability of the Marine Corps operational command to respond effectively to combat and operational stress across the spectrum of stress-problem severity and to maintain troop morale and readiness. OSCAR is innovative in its effort to achieve these goals by integrating modern psychiatric expertise, concepts, and tools into military culture.

In its original conceptualization, OSCAR was expected to do the following (Nash, 2006):

- mitigate stigmatization of mental health problems
- increase knowledge and understanding of the principles of combat stress response and recovery
- improve management of combat stress problems at the small-unit level
- facilitate access to mental health treatment
- prevent and reduce long-term stress and mental health problems.

Overview of the OSCAR Evaluation

To assess the effectiveness of OSCAR in fulfilling its mission, RAND Corporation researchers conducted an evaluation of the OSCAR program that had two primary aims:

1. to determine the impact of OSCAR on proximal and distal outcomes related to combat and operational stress control
2. to determine leadership perceptions of the utility and effectiveness of OSCAR.

Table 1.1 describes these aims and the methods used to accomplish them.

The goal of the first aim was to determine OSCAR's impact on a wide array of proximal (short-term) and distal (long-term) outcomes that the program was designed to target. We achieved this aim by conducting a quasi-experimental study to compare Marines in battalions that received OSCAR training prior to deployment who deployed with a team of OSCAR personnel attached to their units (OSCAR-trained battalions) with Marines in battalions that did not receive OSCAR training prior to deployment (non–OSCAR-trained battalions). Marines in units deploying to Afghanistan or Iraq between March 2010 and December 2011 were surveyed twice, once before (T1) and once after deployment (T2),[1] on a wide array of stress-related attitudes, behaviors, and psychological functioning. Data collection began in March 2010 and concluded in October 2012. This evaluation component, referred to hereafter as the individual Marine survey, is designed to determine whether Marines from OSCAR-trained battalions

Table 1.1
Aims and Methods of the OSCAR Evaluation

Aims	Methods
1. To determine the impact of OSCAR on proximal and distal outcomes related to combat and operational stress control Proximal outcomes • attitudes toward stress response and recovery • perceived support for help-seeking • seeking help for stress and mental health problems from appropriate resources • unit cohesion Distal outcomes • mental health • alcohol use	**Individual Marine survey** Longitudinal pre- (T1) and postdeployment (T2) surveys of 1,307 Marines from OSCAR-trained and non–OSCAR-trained battalions
2. To determine leadership perceptions of OSCAR's impact on • attitudes toward stress response and recovery • unit cohesion and morale • stigma around mental health and help-seeking • unit leaders' abilities to prevent, identify, and manage combat stress problems in the unit	• **Team member survey:** Longitudinal pre- and post-deployment surveys of 91 leaders, medical personnel, and chaplains who attended the OSCAR team member training prior to deployment • **Focus groups:** Focus groups conducted with Marines, primarily small-unit leaders, who had deployed with an OSCAR-trained battalion • **Interviews:** Semistructured interviews conducted with commanding officers of battalions that had received OSCAR training

NOTE: Shorthand labels for the methods used throughout the remainder of this report are indicated in bold type.

---

[1] Throughout the remainder of the report, we refer to pre- and postdeployment surveys as the T1 and T2 surveys, respectively.

fare better on stress-related attitudes and behaviors from pre- to postdeployment than Marines from non–OSCAR-trained battalions.

The goal of the second aim was to determine leadership perceptions of OSCAR's impact on a wide array of outcomes pertinent to combat and operational stress control. This aim was achieved using three methods. First, we conducted an assessment of pre- to postdeployment changes on OSCAR team members' perceptions of the climate around stress response and recovery, as well as OSCAR's impact on this climate and the prevention, identification, and management of combat stress problems. We sampled respondents from the same OSCAR-trained battalions from which individual Marine survey respondents were sampled, and we administered pre- (T1) and postdeployment (T2) surveys at the same time for both of these components. Thus, data collection for the team member survey component also began in March 2010 and ended in October 2012.

We also conducted seven focus groups with Marines from five battalions from December 2010 to June 2012 and 18 interviews with battalion commanding officers of OSCAR-trained battalions in the spring of 2012. Both the focus groups and interviews were designed to gauge leaders' perceptions of the climate around stress response and recovery within their own units and the Marine Corps more broadly, as well as their perceptions of how well OSCAR met the needs of Marines in the prevention, identification, and management of combat and operational stress. The open-ended nature of the questions asked in focus groups and interviews permitted the extraction of richer, more-detailed responses to understand in greater depth how Marines, especially Marine Corps leaders, viewed these topics.

Purpose and Organization of This Report

This report describes the design, findings, and recommendations from this evaluation. As such, this report has utility for policymakers interested in the psychological health of military service members and the effectiveness of military programs designed to prevent, identify, and treat combat and operational stress problems across a range of problem severity.

The remainder of this report is divided into six chapters. In Chapter Two, we provide a detailed description of the history, development, and intended implementation of the OSCAR program, reporting on the methods and results of each of the four evaluation components in four separate chapters. In Chapters Three and Four, we describe findings from the longitudinal T1 and T2 surveys of Marines from OSCAR-trained and non–OSCAR-trained battalions (individual Marine survey) and OSCAR team members (team member survey), respectively. In Chapters Five and Six, we elucidate findings from the focus groups and interviews, respectively. Finally, in Chapter Seven, we integrate findings from the four evaluation components and present our overall conclusions and recommendations for improving the OSCAR program to enhance its effectiveness in the prevention, identification, and treatment of combat and operational stress problems.

CHAPTER TWO

Development and Description of the Operational Stress Control and Readiness Program

In this chapter, we review the history and development of the OSCAR program, provide a detailed description of its conceptualization and intended implementation during the period of this evaluation, and summarize earlier efforts to evaluate it.

History and Development of the OSCAR Program

Within the past decade, DoD has marshaled considerable resources to address combat stress problems experienced by service members returning from the wars in Iraq and Afghanistan. However, military leadership's awareness of and efforts to manage adverse combat stress reactions long predate the wars in Iraq and Afghanistan. Psychiatric treatment for severe combat stress reactions first became an integral part of military medicine during World War I (Shepard, 2001). Since that time, there has been a strong tendency toward a demedicalized approach to problems of combat stress. This approach favors group cohesion, peer support, treatment close to the front lines when necessary, and rapid return to action for affected combatants over more-intensive medical treatments that require removal of affected combatants from their units (Nash, 2006; Office of the Inspector General, 1996). However, integrating the operational and medical priorities into effective systems for managing operational stress remains a significant military policy challenge (Wessely, 2006).

The first attempts to integrate the psychiatric and operational approaches to combat stress reaction were made toward the end of World War I under the banner of "forward psychiatry," a program of positioning psychiatric care immediately behind the front lines to avoid the need for evacuation of psychiatric casualties. The principles of forward psychiatry were captured in the acronym PIE: proximity, immediacy, and expectancy. *Proximity* refers to management of combat stress problems in or "as near as possible to the battle line" (Office of the Inspector General, 1996, p. 13). The principle of immediacy underscores the importance of managing combat stress problems as soon as they have been recognized. The principle of expectancy highlights the importance of positive expectations for recovery; service members should be taught that the most likely outcome of combat stress injury is a quick and full recovery.

In 1996, the Office of the Inspector General published an evaluation of DoD's efforts to manage and mitigate combat stress during previous wars, highlighting the importance of the PIE principles. This report recommended that all branches of service develop and implement their own operational stress–control programs and that these programs be comprehensive, meaning that they should address prevention of combat stress reactions, early identification of combat stress reactions when they occur, and effective treatment for those in need. These recommendations were released in DoD Directive 6490.5 to all branches of service to establish comprehensive operational stress–control programs in 1999 (Assistant Secretary of Defense for Health Affairs, 1999).

The Marine Corps had a combat stress–control program at that time, but it was neither comprehensive nor well integrated into the operational command structure. The program included three surgical companies, each with its own combat stress platoon made up of one psychiatrist, two psychologists, and three psychology technicians (Office of the Inspector General, 1996). Services were located at a distance from the front lines of combat. The OSCAR program, established as part of the Marine Corps' response to the 1999 DoD directive, aimed to create a "new type of partnership between warfighters and mental health professionals" (Nash, 2006, p. 25-6) that would enable "prevention, early identification, and effective treatment [of combat and operational stress problems] *at the lowest level possible*" (Nash, 2006, p. 25-6). The OSCAR program was first established in 1999 in the 2nd Marine Division, based in Camp Lejeune, North Carolina.

OSCAR's Goals

OSCAR aims to bridge the medical/operational divide in both directions, bringing mental health clinicians into the context of combat operations and familiarizing operational leaders with basic clinical understandings of combat stress. Psychiatrists, psychologists, and psychological technicians are positioned within operational units as part of OSCAR teams so that they become organic to those units, similar to surgeons, corpsmen, and chaplains. The OSCAR teams are expected to participate with their Marines in predeployment training, go with them into forward operational areas during deployment, and continue in a supportive role after their Marines return from deployment. In addition to being immediately accessible when needed, clinicians would be better equipped to understand and provide authoritative counseling to Marines in crisis because of their shared experiences.

At the same time, OSCAR also involves training for non–mental health professionals, including chaplains, corpsmen, and select NCOs and officers at the battalion and company levels, in the identification of emerging combat stress–related mental health problems. The NCOs and officers, who are ultimately responsible for combat and operational stress control within the units they lead, typically have the earliest opportunity to identify and address combat stress problems in Marines. In most cases, the NCOs and officers should be able to assist these Marines by helping to marshal informal sources of peer support. In cases in which clinical intervention is required, the NCOs and officers are in the best position to make a timely and appropriate referral. The OSCAR training for NCOs and officers was designed to give them the skills to make these triage decisions.

OSCAR's Evolution

Since its inception in 1999, OSCAR has grown and evolved as it has gained traction with Marine Corps leadership. In 2003, the medical officer of the Marine Corps promoted the implementation of OSCAR in all three active-component Marine Corps infantry divisions (Nash, 2006), which was initiated in January 2004 as a two-year pilot of the OSCAR program. In 2006, the Army released a revised version (Headquarters Department of the Army, 2006) of the combat and operational stress–control doctrine that was distributed to all of the branches of service in 1999 in DoD Directive 6490.5 (Assistant Secretary of Defense for Health Affairs, 1999). Both the Navy and Marine Corps disagreed with the Army's revised doctrine and, in response, developed their own combat and operational stress–control doctrine[1] in 2007 that was foundational but not unique to OSCAR (Chief of Naval Operations and Commandant of the Marine Corps , 2010). In 2007, the Commanding Generals of all three Marine Expeditionary Forces (MEFs) collectively requested that HQMC and Navy Medicine institutionalize, staff, and support OSCAR (Chief of Naval Operations and Commandant of the Marine Corps, 2010). In 2008, the Marine Corps Development Command and the Chief of Naval Personnel prioritized the allocation of personnel for OSCAR to ensure its permanence, granting a total of 26 positions for mental health professionals and 29 positions for paraprofessional psychiatric technician corpsmen in Marine Corps infantry divisions and regiments of the active and reserve components to be filled by 2011 (Weinick et al., 2011). In 2009, under direction of the Assistant Commandant of the Marine Corps, OSCAR capabilities were extended down to the battalion and company levels without the provision of additional mental health professionals (Weinick et al., 2011). This extension was accomplished by adding medical and religious ministry personnel and select NCOs and officers at the battalion and company levels. Additional training in the prevention, identification, and treatment of combat stress problems was provided to select NCOs and officers to prepare them for their role on the OSCAR team. In October 2011, the Deputy Commandant for Manpower and Reserve Affairs of the Marine Corps released a Marine Administrative Message (MARADMIN) requiring Marine Corps–wide dissemination of the OSCAR program, i.e., the formation of OSCAR teams and provision of OSCAR training in all "battalion-level or equivalent commands across the total force" by January 31, 2012 (U.S. Marine Corps, 2011).

Description of the OSCAR Program

Our description of the OSCAR program is focused on its conceptualization and intended implementation during the period of data collection for the OSCAR evaluation, March 2010 through October 2012. During this period, the OSCAR program was driven largely by the training provided to the three types of OSCAR personnel: team members, extenders, and mental health professionals. As depicted in the logic model of OSCAR (see Figure 2.1), the goal of the training was to better manage combat stress during deployment through improved prevention and resilience, access to care, and operational effectiveness. These outcomes are meant to occur through the actions of people trained to identify combat stress problems and react quickly and appropriately, as well as through reduction in the stigma attached to combat stress reactions and mental health care. Improved management of combat stress during deployment is expected to have a positive effect on long-term outcomes of interest, including better mental health, lower levels of alcohol use, and lower levels of impairment in work productivity.

Below we describe the different types of personnel who play a role in implementing the OSCAR program. We also provide additional details about the format and content of the OSCAR team member training course, including its underlying theoretical framework, and highlight the innovative aspects of OSCAR relative to other components of the HQMC combat and operational stress–control program.

---

[1] We describe the combat and operational stress–control doctrine endorsed by the Navy and Marine Corps in greater detail later in this chapter in the section titled "Theoretical Framework Underlying OSCAR Training."

Figure 2.1
OSCAR Logic Model

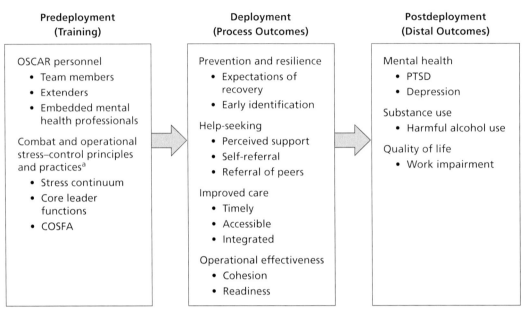

NOTE: COSFA = Combat and Operational Stress First Aid. PTSD = posttraumatic stress disorder.
[a] Combat and operational stress–control principles and practices are presented in OSCAR training but are not unique to OSCAR. Rather, they are broadly endorsed by both the Marine Corps and Navy and are presented to Marines in multiple venues.
RAND RR562-2.1

OSCAR Personnel

According to the most recently released guidance on the OSCAR program (U.S. Marine Corps, 2011), the OSCAR program made use of five types of people:

1. *OSCAR providers* are mental health care professionals embedded in Marine Corps infantry units at the regiment and division levels. OSCAR providers are available in theater to support the mental health needs of Marines. In addition to providing clinical services, OSCAR providers are expected to have regular interactions with the unit in a variety of nonclinical capacities to help Marines become familiar with the providers and to ensure the providers' awareness and understanding of mission requirements.

2. *OSCAR extenders* are selected physicians (other than psychiatrists), dental officers, nurses, other medical service providers, chaplains, religious program specialists, and corpsmen attached at the battalion and company levels. These people are expected to mitigate and manage the stress problems of Marines referred to them by unit leaders and, when the problems exceed their skill levels, make referrals to OSCAR providers.

3. *OSCAR team members*, sometimes referred to as OSCAR mentors, are officers and NCOs at the battalion and company levels who have been selected by their unit commanding officers on the basis of their perceived ability to lead effectively, serve as positive role models, and help and mentor Marines with stress problems. OSCAR team members are intended to be first responders for Marines experiencing combat and operational stress. Relative to OSCAR providers or extenders, OSCAR team members are close to the field and the small-unit level, giving them the earliest opportunity to identify a Marine

in distress and support Marines who are showing signs of distress. The support they provide includes assistance with mitigation of controllable stressors, psychological first aid for Marines experiencing acute stress reactions, referrals to OSCAR extenders or providers for treatment of more-severe stress problems, and facilitation of reintegration into the unit after treatment for severe stress problems. OSCAR team members are also expected to mitigate stigma around seeking help for stress and mental health problems.

4. An *OSCAR trainer* is a Marine who has successfully completed a five-day train-the-trainer course conducted by an OSCAR master trainer. OSCAR master trainers certify OSCAR trainers throughout the force to ensure a sufficient supply of OSCAR trainers who can train units across the total force.

5. An *OSCAR master trainer* is a Marine who has successfully completed a seven-day course and received certification to train OSCAR trainers from personnel at HQMC Combat and Operational Stress Control (COSC). Personnel from HQMC COSC provide training as OSCAR master trainers at regular intervals at each of the MEFs and the Marine Corps Forces Reserve Headquarters to ensure a sufficient supply of qualified OSCAR master trainers.

The first three types of people—OSCAR providers, extenders, and team members— form an OSCAR team whose purpose is to prevent, identify, and treat combat stress problems experienced by the Marines in their units. Per the HQMC mandate that each battalion in the Marine Corps assemble and train an OSCAR team by January 31, 2012 (U.S. Marine Corps, 2011), each battalion's OSCAR team must consist of a minimum of 5 percent of the battalion's personnel or 20 Marines and sailors, whichever is greater. The NCOs and officers constitute the majority of the OSCAR team.

OSCAR Team Member Training

OSCAR team member training is conducted as part of a battalion's deployment preparations three to five months before deployment. The training is conducted at the battalion level in an interactive group presentation format by OSCAR trainers. Typically, the OSCAR training is delivered during a single day and lasts from morning until midafternoon. Training is geared primarily toward the battalion's OSCAR team members, but OSCAR extenders and providers are also expected to attend.

The group sessions include an overview of the objectives of the OSCAR program, information on the biological basis of stress reactions and their social and behavioral impacts on soldiers, implications for mission readiness among soldiers and units, and the ways in which the OSCAR program seeks to improve management of combat stress. The trainers also lead group discussions and conduct role-playing exercises designed to help the officers and NCOs practice the skill sets important for preventing, identifying, and managing stress problems among Marines. The training concludes with a panel of experienced Marines who share their own experiences with combat stress and discuss how the principles of the OSCAR program apply to them. OSCAR team members are expected to employ the skills covered in the training both during and after a deployment, though the biggest impact of the training on a particular battalion is likely to be felt during a deployment.

The OSCAR training curriculum is outlined in a manual created by HQMC COSC. Per the OSCAR training guidance that HQMC released in October 2011 (U.S. Marine Corps, 2011), OSCAR trainers should maintain fidelity to the curriculum in the manual. However,

OSCAR trainers are encouraged to tailor the training to the unit by, for instance, generating examples that will resonate with group participants and modifying the presentation slides to display the local command logo and OSCAR structure. As with any program, some variation in the implementation of OSCAR across units is to be expected. Based on anecdotal reports from our points of contact in the units from which participants in various components of this evaluation were selected, there appears to have been wide variation in the implementation of OSCAR. For example, the point of contact for one unit reported that predeployment OSCAR team member training had been conducted with roughly half of the battalion, including junior enlisted Marines. In contrast, Marines in another unit who participated in focus groups reported that OSCAR team member training for their units consisted of a 30-minute briefing. However, the extent and nature of variation in the implementation of OSCAR across the Marine Corps are unknown.

Theoretical Framework Underlying OSCAR Training

The theoretical framework that underlies OSCAR training is the same framework that underlies both the Marine Corps' and Navy's comprehensive combat and operational stress–control programs. The cornerstone of their approach to control combat and operational stress is the Combat and Operational Stress Continuum model (hereafter referred to as the stress-continuum model), a tool for identifying combat stress problems of varying severity. Built on the stress continuum model are two interrelated sets of prescribed actions to prevent and treat combat stress problems of varying severity: (1) the five core leader functions and (2) a psychological first aid intervention adapted for combat and operational stress, COSFA.

The OSCAR training course is designed to provide education and practice in implementing the combat and operational stress–control principles embodied in the stress-continuum model, the five core leader functions, and COSFA. However, these principles are not unique to OSCAR: All leaders in the U.S. Marine Corps (USMC) and Navy are expected to know and practice these principles of combat and operational stress control.

The stress-continuum model, five core leader functions, and COSFA are described in detail in Appendix A. Next, we summarize the available empirical evidence relevant to this theoretical framework.

Evidence Base for the Theoretical Framework Underlying OSCAR

The developers of the theoretical framework that undergirds the Marine Corps' and Navy's current combat and operational stress–control doctrine, including the principles of the OSCAR program and its attendant tools—the stress-continuum model, core leader functions, and COSFA—endeavored to incorporate the best available scientific evidence to conceptualize OSCAR (Nash, 2011; Nash, Krantz, et al., 2011). However, they readily acknowledge that the tools of the program lack empirical evidence of their effectiveness in the prevention, identification, and treatment of combat stress reactions, injuries, and illnesses (Nash, 2011; Nash, Krantz, et al., 2011). Moreover, the psychological first aid techniques on which COSFA is based are themselves merely evidence-informed, as opposed to evidence-based; no empirical support of their effectiveness at preventing the development and escalation of mental health problems has yet been demonstrated.

These caveats notwithstanding, many of the interventions that make up OSCAR, including psychological first aid, are recommended by expert consensus as described in the U.S. Department of Veterans Affairs/DoD Clinical Practice Guidelines on the management of acute stress and interventions to prevent PTSD (Nash and Watson, 2012). Thus, although the combat and operational stress–control doctrine that is the foundation for OSCAR was not based on empirical evidence, because such evidence was lacking, it was based on the best information available at the time of its development.

The paucity of empirical evidence of effectiveness is not limited to the tools outlined in combat and operational stress–control doctrine. Indeed, a recent RAND review of resilience programs in DoD concluded that there was no evidence of the effectiveness of any of the DoD resilience programs in preventing future mental health problems (Meredith et al., 2011). Similarly, a recently released Institute of Medicine (IOM) review of the treatment of PTSD in military and veteran populations concluded that there are no evidence-based approaches to the prevention of PTSD (IOM, 2014). Thus, the promise of DoD resilience programs has yet to be empirically realized.

OSCAR in the Context of HQMC Combat and Operational Stress Control

To understand the OSCAR program, it is essential to understand where it fits in the broader landscape of the Marine Corps' comprehensive COSC program, of which OSCAR is just one—albeit one very important—component. The principles and theoretical framework on which OSCAR is based are those of the Marine Corps' comprehensive COSC program, and OSCAR is not the only venue in which the Marine Corps communicates its policies and principles regarding combat and operational stress. All Marines attend COSC training in career school and for any deployment that lasts for at least 90 days (Meredith et al., 2011). Deployment-cycle training briefs are delivered within 30 days before deployment (Warrior Preparation), within seven days of redeployment (Warrior Transition), and 60 to 90 days after redeployment (Warrior Transition–II) (Nash, Krantz, et al., 2011). In addition, the principles of the COSC program are disseminated to high-risk families of Marines who have undergone multiple deployments with a high operational tempo through the Families OverComing Under Stress (FOCUS) program operated by the Navy Bureau of Medicine and Surgery (Weinick et al., 2011).[2]

Clearly, then, the principles of combat and operational stress control imparted during the OSCAR training course do not distinguish OSCAR in its current conceptualization from other COSC efforts. What does appear to make OSCAR unique within the broader context of the HQMC COSC program are the distinctive, formalized roles assigned to the people in the unit who form the OSCAR team (i.e., OSCAR providers, extenders, and team members); the emphasis on coordination and collaboration among the people on the OSCAR team; and, harkening back to the original motivation behind OSCAR's genesis, the integration of mental health professionals and modern psychiatric concepts and tools into military culture.

Previous Evaluations of OSCAR

The OSCAR evaluation on which this report centers is not the first effort to evaluate OSCAR. The first effort to evaluate OSCAR was a small, unpublished study that focused on the two-year pilot project in which OSCAR was implemented across all three active Marine Corps

---

[2] The FOCUS program is designed to increase family resiliency and targets high-risk families in all branches of service, not just the Marine Corps.

divisions (MARDIVs) (personal communication with HQMC official, 2009). The findings suggested that OSCAR had performed well enough to warrant more-widespread dissemination to wing and logistic units and the Marine Corps Reserve but that it should continue to be evaluated to ensure that it fulfilled its potential. The findings further suggested that there was considerable variability in the implementation of OSCAR across the three MARDIVs and OSCAR providers and that coordination of OSCAR with other HQMC COSC programs should be improved.

In addition, RAND researchers observed the first OSCAR team member training, which took place on January 21, 2010, at the Marine Corps base in Twenty-Nine Palms, California, to evaluate the effectiveness of newly redesigned training materials. To evaluate the training, the RAND team administered a pre- and posttraining survey designed to assess changes in training attendees' knowledge, preparedness, and confidence to employ the skills covered in OSCAR training. In general, OSCAR team members reported positive perceptions of the training experience, although the RAND team identified some areas of concern with respect to OSCAR's potential to affect help-seeking behavior. These areas of concern included team members' abilities to facilitate unit reintegration of Marines who had been treated for stress problems and awareness of resources available to help Marines cope with stress experienced in theater and in garrison. The evaluation also revealed some potential challenges to OSCAR's success, including team members' perceptions that their chains of command might not acknowledge the importance of combat and operational stress control, that Marines who discuss their levels of stress control will have concerns about stigmatization, and that Marines will be concerned about confidentiality when discussing their stress levels with OSCAR team members. The report documenting the findings from this evaluation is reproduced in Appendix B.

Summary

In summary, the OSCAR program was originally conceived of as a new partnership between psychiatry and the military. At the inception of OSCAR, this partnership was implemented by embedding mental health professionals at the regiment level to integrate them into military culture. Over time, OSCAR has evolved to extend the capabilities of OSCAR providers down to the battalion and company levels by adding to the OSCAR team medical and religious ministry personnel (OSCAR extenders) and select NCOs and officers (OSCAR team members) who have received training in combat and operational stress–control principles and practices. The theoretical model on which OSCAR team member training is based is the same theoretical model that underlies the Marine Corps' comprehensive COSC program. This model is made up of related sets of principles and skills for preventing, identifying, and managing combat and operational stress problems, including the stress continuum, the five core leader functions, and COSFA. At present, OSCAR is distinctive from other Marine Corps COSC efforts in its emphasis on formally assigned roles (OSCAR providers, extenders, and team members) to different types of people in the unit and collaboration among these people to bring the tools and concepts of modern psychiatry closer to the front lines of combat and thus improve combat and operational stress control.

CHAPTER THREE

Evaluation of OSCAR's Impact on Help-Seeking and Mental Health: Individual Marine Survey

Although OSCAR gained enough traction with Marine Corps leadership to be disseminated throughout the Marine Corps, its effectiveness at improving combat stress–related outcomes had not been tested. To address this gap, we evaluated its impact on a wide array of short- and long-term outcomes. The short-term outcomes included attitudes and behaviors directly targeted by the OSCAR training, such as help-seeking for stress-related problems. Long-term outcomes included aspects of health and well-being that might be improved if positive changes in short-term outcomes resulted in longer-term sustained benefits (e.g., if better help-seeking increased mental health care use, which, in turn, led to improved symptoms). The design of the study was quasi-experimental; a comparison was made between Marines who deployed in battalions that had OSCAR-trained teams (OSCAR-trained battalions, i.e., intervention group) and Marines who deployed with battalions that did not have OSCAR-trained teams (non–OSCAR-trained battalions, i.e., control group), but there was no random assignment to the intervention or control groups. This chapter summarizes the methods and results of this evaluation component and concludes with a discussion of its implications and limitations. A more detailed description of the sampling strategy, procedures, measures, and statistical analysis can be found in Appendix C.

Methods

Sampling

The sampling procedure consisted of two stages: (1) sampling eligible battalions and (2) sampling companies within each of the selected battalions. Our contacts in the HQMC COSC office identified OSCAR-trained and non–OSCAR-trained battalions that were active-duty or reserve units preparing for a combat deployment to Iraq or Afghanistan in 2010 or 2011. In the first stage, we sampled six battalions scheduled to receive OSCAR training—four infantry battalions and two combat service–support battalions (i.e., combat logistics and engineering support battalions)—and two control battalions,[1] both of which were service-support battalions.

In the second stage, companies were sampled from within the selected battalions. Given variability in the organization of battalions and their ability to coordinate the survey, the procedure for sampling companies varied across battalions, and thus the number of Marines per

---

[1] Because of a MARADMIN released from HQMC in October 2011 that mandated dissemination of OSCAR to all battalions in the Marine Corps by January 31, 2012, we had difficulty identifying for the control group those battalions that had not received OSCAR training. Thus, our sample size for the control group is roughly half of the intervention group's sample size.

sampled battalion varied as well. All Marines of rank O6 (colonel) or lower within each company were asked to complete the T1 survey. Only those Marines who subsequently deployed to Iraq or Afghanistan are included in the present analysis.[2]

A total of 2,975 Marines were asked to complete the T1 survey.[3] Of these Marines, 2,620 (88 percent) completed the T1[4] survey, and 2,523 subsequently deployed to Iraq or Afghanistan. Among the 2,523 Marines, 1,631 were in battalions that received OSCAR training, and 892 were in battalions that did not receive OSCAR training (see Appendix C for technical details on the computation of the survey response rate).

Procedures

Data collection took place between March 2010 and October 2012. For the T1 survey, pencil-and-paper self-report surveys were administered in a group setting on base by a survey administrator outside the chain of command, i.e., COSC or RAND personnel or the unit chaplain or religious program specialist. For respondents in OSCAR-trained battalions, T1 surveys were administered prior to the battalion's OSCAR training to obtain a baseline assessment of the outcomes of interest. Respondents were informed that participation was voluntary and that their responses would be kept confidential. Written informed consent was obtained. The amount of time between the date of the T1 survey administration and deployment varied across battalions, with an average of 61.1 days (standard deviation [SD] = 46.8 days) between these dates (minimum: 13 days; maximum: 6.5 months).

We aimed to administer the T2 survey to all T1 survey completers in a group setting on base approximately two to three months after redeployment from Iraq or Afghanistan. The lag between redeployment and the T2 assessment was intended to permit the passage of enough time for serious long-term mental health and functioning outcomes to become apparent. On average, the length of time between the dates of the unit's redeployment and the T2 survey was 92.2 days (SD = 3.4 months), with considerable variability (minimum: four days; maximum: 17.5 months). Variation in the length of time between redeployment and the T2 assessment was taken into account in the statistical analysis.

Of the 2,523 eligible Marines who completed the T1, 51.8 percent also completed the T2 survey, resulting in a final sample size of 1,307. Only a small percentage of T1 survey completers explicitly refused to complete the T2 survey ($n = 194$, 7.7 percent). Rather, most Marines who did not complete the T2 survey simply could not be located after redeployment because of permanent change of station (PCS) or end of active service (EAS). When a Marine was not present at the on-base T2 survey administration and a home address was available ($n = 717$), we mailed the T2 survey to his or her home address in an effort to maximize the study retention rate, although only 61 (8.5 percent) returned completed surveys.

---

[2]   A secondary analysis of T1 survey data was conducted, and the findings and recommendations from this analysis are described in a separate report (Farmer et al., 2014). The secondary analysis made use of available data on all T1 survey respondents ($N = 2,620$), not just those who were eligible for inclusion in this analysis.

[3]   This number underestimates the number of Marines who could have participated in the study. There might have been other Marines in the units targeted for the survey who were eligible to participate and passively refused by not returning their surveys or returning them blank without explicitly indicating their refusal to participate on the survey. In the absence of returned surveys with marking to acknowledge the decision to participate (or not), we do not know whether those Marines had the opportunity to participate in the survey.

[4]   A total of 355 Marines explicitly declined to participate in the T1 survey.

To assess the possible impact of attrition on the final sample composition, we conducted cluster-adjusted Wald chi-square tests of significance to compare the T2 survey completers (n = 1,307) and noncompleters (n = 1,216) on all of the sociodemographic and service history characteristics and baseline levels of the outcomes of interest measured in the T1 survey (see Table 3.1 for a list of outcomes measured in the T1 survey). The two groups differed significantly on parental status and deployment history.[5] Marines who did not complete the T2 survey were more likely to have children and to have deployed previously to Iraq or Afghanistan at least once.

Measures

The T1 and T2 surveys were nearly identical in content so that changes over time could be assessed. Information was also collected on factors that might have confounded OSCAR's effects, including sociodemographic and service history characteristics, lifetime history of traumatic events, deployment experiences, and baseline levels of the outcomes of interest.[6] Outcomes of interest included expectancies regarding stress response and recovery, perceived support for help-seeking, support- and help-seeking behavior, unit support, current stress levels, probable PTSD, probable major depressive disorder (MDD), high-risk alcohol use, general health, and occupational functioning.

We selected well-validated measures of the constructs of interest where available. For several outcomes, however, either measures had been used in previous studies but not extensively validated or measures did not exist. In these instances, we borrowed relevant items from surveys and, when this was not possible, developed new survey items to capture the construct of interest. Measures of individual characteristics, deployment experiences, and outcomes are summarized in Table 3.1. More-detailed descriptions of these measures, including previous research on their psychometric properties and how they were scored for this analysis, are available in Appendix C.

Statistical Analysis

To evaluate OSCAR's impact on the outcomes of interest, we conducted difference-in-differences analyses in which we compared Marines in the OSCAR-trained and non–OSCAR-trained battalions on pre- to postdeployment differences in key outcomes. Analyses included a series of regression models in which we estimated the association of OSCAR with differences over time in key outcomes. Because the study design was quasi-experimental (i.e., battalions received OSCAR training at the discretion of Marine Corps leadership rather than having an equal chance of receiving OSCAR as the result of random assignment[7]) and Marines in the OSCAR-trained and control battalions differed on several potentially confounding baseline

---

[5] Tests of significance and descriptive statistics on the variables on which differences were found were as follows: The two groups differed significantly only on parental status (Wald chi-square = 7.58, p = 0.01) and deployment history (Wald chi-square = 5.79, p = 0.03). Marines who did not complete the T2 survey were more likely to have one or more children (noncompleters: 24.0 percent parents; completers: 19.8 percent parents) and to have deployed previously to Iraq or Afghanistan at least once (noncompleters: 50.4 percent previously deployed; completers: 34.1 percent previously deployed).

[6] Sex was not assessed on the survey because of concerns that this would greatly increase the risk of identifiability of female survey respondents because women constitute a very small proportion of Marines.

[7] At the inception of data collection in March 2010, infantry units received priority for OSCAR training over service-support units, such as combat logistics and engineering support battalions.

Table 3.1
Measures of Individual Characteristics, Deployment Experiences, and Outcomes

Construct	Measure Description	Measure Title and Citation	T1 Survey	T2 Survey
Individual characteristics and deployment experiences				
Sociodemographic and service history characteristics	Items assessing • rank • age • race or ethnicity • marital status • number of children • number of previous deployments to Iraq or Afghanistan • number of stress classes attended prior to or since joining one's current unit	Items were created for this study	X	
	Administrative data on • number of days between the T1 survey administration and the date of deployment • number of days between the T2 survey administration and the date of redeployment	N/A—administrative data		
Lifetime history of potentially traumatic events	List of 17 types of potentially traumatic events; respondents indicate which of these events they have directly experienced in their lifetimes	Life Events Checklist (LEC) (Gray et al., 2004)	X	
Combat experiences during deployment	List of 10 types of combat experiences rated on the frequency with which they occurred during the most recent deployment	Combat Experiences subscale of the Deployment Risk and Resilience Inventory (DRRI) (King et al., 2006; Vogt et al., 2008)		X
Peritraumatic distress	15 items assessing the severity of distress and dissociation experienced at the time of the most stressful experience of the most recent deployment	Peritraumatic Behavior Questionnaire—Self-Rated version (PBQ-SR) (Nash, Goldwasser, et al., 2009)		X
Deployment environment	20 items assessing the frequency of irritations and discomfort experienced during the most recent deployment	DRRI Difficulty Living and Working Environment subscale (King et al., 2006)		X
Proximal outcomes				
Expectancies regarding stress response and recovery	13 items assessing beliefs about responding to and recovering from stress problems	Measure was created for this study	X	X
Perceived support for help-seeking	10 items assessing perceived support from other Marines for seeking help for stress problems	Measure was created for this study	X	X
Support-seeking behavior[a]	Utilization of a fellow Marine or leader for help with one's stress Recommendation of a fellow Marine or leader to a peer for help with stress	Measure was created for this study		
Help-seeking behavior	Utilization of one of the following resources for help with one's own stress • chaplain • corpsman • unit medical officer	Measure was created for this study	X	X

Table 3.1—Continued

Construct	Measure Description	Measure Title and Citation	T1 Survey	T2 Survey
Help-seeking behavior, continued	Recommending one of the following resources to a fellow Marine for help with his or her (Marine's) stress • chaplain • corpsman • unit medical officer	Measure was created for this study.	X	X
Unit support	12 items assessing perceived support (generally, not specifically for stress) from the military in general, unit leaders, and other unit members	Deployment Social Support subscale of the DRRI (King et al., 2006)	X	X
Distal outcomes				
Current stress levels	Single-item self-rating of one's current zone on the Combat and Operational Stress Continuum	Measure was created for this study	X	X
PTSD	17 items assessing the severity of PTSD symptoms experienced over the course of a lifetime	Modified version[b] of the Post-Traumatic Symptom Checklist–Civilian version (PCL-C) (Weathers, Huska, and Keane, 1991)	X	
	17 items assessing the severity of PTSD symptoms experienced in the past month and used to determine current probable PTSD via the cluster scoring method	Standard PCL-C (Weathers, Huska, and Keane, 1991)		X
MDD	2-item screener for MDD, modified from the standard time frame of past 2 weeks to past month for the current study	Patient Health Questionnaire–2 (PHQ-2) (Kroenke, Spitzer, and Williams, 2003)	X	
	8-item measure of the frequency of depressive symptoms experienced in the past 2 weeks; current probable MDD determined by symptom severity score of 10 or higher	Patient Health Questionnaire–8 (PHQ-8) (Kroenke, Spitzer, and Williams, 2001; Löwe et al., 2004)		X
High-risk alcohol use	3-item measure of the quantity and frequency of alcohol consumption; positive screen for high-risk alcohol use indicated by a score of 8 or higher	Alcohol Use Disorders Identification Test–Consumption (AUDIT-C) (Bush et al., 1998)	X	X
General health	Single-item assessment of one's overall general health	Short-Form Health Survey (SF-12) (Ware, Kosinski, and Keller, 1996)	X	X
Occupational impairment	5-item measure of the frequency of impairment experienced on the job in the past 4 weeks	Health Performance Questionnaire (HPQ) (Kessler et al., 2003)	X	X

[a] We use the term *support-seeking* to refer to seeking help for stress from a fellow Marine or leader to distinguish these informal sources of help from more-formal sources of help, such as chaplains, corpsmen, and unit medical officers. This distinction is used in an effort to be consistent with the broader literature on *help-seeking*, which typically refers to seeking help for mental health problems from formal sources of support, such as mental health care providers.

[b] The time frame for reporting symptoms on the PCL-C in the T1 survey was modified from the standard time frame of "past 30 days" to lifetime.

characteristics and deployment experiences, it was necessary to adjust statistically for these group differences. We adjusted for these differences with a doubly robust method that included propensity score weighting and the inclusion of baseline characteristics and deployment experiences as predictors in the regression model. All of the individual characteristics, deployment experiences, and baseline levels of the outcomes listed in Table 3.1 were included both as predictors in the models estimated to create propensity score weights and as covariates in the multivariate regression models estimating OSCAR's impact on outcomes. All multivariate models also adjusted for the clustering of participants within battalions.

The method of recycled predictions was used to translate the model results into the predicted prevalence of each outcome with and without OSCAR training (Graubard and Korn, 1999; Setodji et al., 2012). This analysis provides our best estimate of the effect of the OSCAR program on the outcomes. The statistical test associated with this effect estimate indicates whether the effect is likely to be due to chance or to the effect of the program; a statistically significant effect estimate indicates a likely effect of OSCAR on an outcome, while a nonsignificant effect estimate indicates that we did not find evidence of an effect of OSCAR on that outcome. In addition to the effect estimate, we also provide the 95-percent confidence interval (CI) for the effect estimate, which is the range in which the true effect is 95 percent likely to lie. We also conducted two sets of sensitivity analyses to examine the extent to which the results were biased by missing data and to disentangle the impact of OSCAR from the primary confound of battalion type (infantry versus service support).[8] Our approach to each of these analyses is described in Appendix C.

Results

In this section, we present descriptive statistics on the final sample of participants ($N = 1,307$), followed by findings from the multivariate regression models that were estimated to determine OSCAR's impact on the outcomes it was designed to target.

Sociodemographic and Service History Characteristics of the Final Sample at Baseline

As shown in Table 3.2, the Marines in the final sample were predominantly younger than 25 years old, white, junior enlisted (rank E1–E3), unmarried, and childless. Roughly two-thirds of the Marines in the sample had never deployed (i.e., they were preparing for their first deployments at the time of this survey), and just over half were in infantry, as opposed to service-support battalions. Given the high representation of younger, lower-ranking Marines, both of which are characteristics associated with greater risk of mental health problems (Brewin, Andrews, and Valentine, 2000; Farmer et al., 2014), our sample includes a high proportion of people who stand to benefit most from programs that, like OSCAR, are aimed at preventing, identifying, and treating stress and mental health problems. A comparison of the sociodemographic and service history characteristics of the final sample and those of the broader popula-

---

[8]   Because the type of battalion (infantry versus service support) was so highly confounded with treatment group (OSCAR-trained versus control battalion), we were unable to include it as a predictor in models to create propensity scores or in multivariate regression models to estimate OSCAR's impact on outcomes. In an attempt to disentangle OSCAR's effects from that of battalion type, we performed a sensitivity analysis to examine OSCAR's impact on outcomes among the subset of Marines in service-support battalions and to determine whether the pattern of findings obtained in the full sample could be replicated.

Table 3.2
Descriptive Statistics of Marines in the Final Sample and in OSCAR-Trained and Control Battalions on Baseline Characteristics and Deployment Experiences

Characteristic or Variable	Entire Sample (N = 1,307)	Control (n = 468)	OSCAR-Trained (n = 839)
Covariates and baseline levels of outcomes assessed in the T1 survey			
		Percentage	
Rank†			
E1–E3	70	58	77
E4–E9	26	36	20
Officer	4	6	3
Age 25 or older*	22	30	17
Race or ethnicity			
White	70	68	72
Black	7	10	5
Hispanic	19	18	19
Other	4	4	4
Married	30	33	29
Has one child or more†	20	23	18
History of at least one deployment at baseline	34	28	37
Infantry (versus service support) battalion[a]	57	0	89
Number of stress classes attended at baseline			
0	12	4	17
1–3	39	36	41
4 or more	49	61	43
Lifetime history of potentially traumatic events			
Sexual assault or other unwanted sexual experience*	6	8	5
Witnessed violent death or experienced sudden, unexpected death of loved one*	50	46	52
Caused serious injury or death of another*	17	10	21
Use of social resources for help with stress problems			
Fellow Marine	75	77	74
Leader*	50	56	46
Chaplain	20	25	17
Corpsman*	23	18	26

Table 3.2—Continued

Characteristic or Variable	Entire Sample (*N* = 1,307)	Control (*n* = 468)	OSCAR-Trained (*n* = 839)
Unit medical officer	11	11	12
Any*[b]	82	86	80
Recommended resources to peer for help with stress problems			
Fellow Marine	85	87	84
Leader*	67	73	64
Chaplain*	56	66	51
Corpsman	38	31	42
Unit medical officer	26	28	25
Any*[b]	90	93	89
		M (SE)	
Expectancies regarding stress response and recovery[c]	4.0 (0.01)	4.0 (0.02)	4.0 (0.02)
Perceived support for help-seeking[d]	3.1 (0.02)	3.2 (0.03)	3.1 (0.02)
Deployment experiences assessed in T2 survey			
		M (SE)	
Combat experiences during deployment†[e]	10.9 (0.89)	9.4 (0.45)	11.8 (1.3)
Deployment environment*[f]	59.1 (2.0)	54.1 (0.90)	62.0 (1.8)

NOTE: All estimates and tests of significance referenced above adjust for clustering of Marines within battalions. Wald chi-squared tests of significance were conducted to compare the Marines in OSCAR-trained and control battalions on all of the variables in the table. M = mean. SE = standard error.

* Statistically significant differences between OSCAR-trained and control battalions at *p* < 0.05.

† Statistical comparisons with a *p*-value less than 0.10 but greater than 0.05. For some variables, the percentages sum to more than 100 because of rounding error.

[a] The significance test to compare the proportions of Marines in OSCAR-trained and control battalions who were sampled from infantry versus service-support battalions could not be computed because there were no infantry battalions in the control group.

[b] *Any* resource used or recommended to a fellow Marine for help with stress problems refers to having used or recommended one or more of the five resources: fellow Marine, leader, chaplain, corpsman, or unit medical officer.

[c] Expectancies regarding stress response and recovery were measured on a scale on which possible scores range from 1 to 5, where higher scores indicate more-positive, healthier expectancies regarding stress response and recovery.

[d] Perceived support for help-seeking was measured on a scale on which possible scores range from 1 to 5, where higher scores indicate greater perceived support for help-seeking.

[e] Combat experiences during deployment were assessed on a scale that ranges from 0 to 40, where higher scores indicate more-frequent exposure to more types of combat experiences.

[f] Deployment environment was measured on a scale on which possible scores range from 20 to 100, where higher scores indicate greater levels of irritation and discomfort experienced during the respondent's most recent deployment.

tion of active and reservist Marines of rank O6 or lower who deployed to Iraq or Afghanistan in 2010 or 2011 is available in Table C.1 in Appendix C.

We compared Marines in OSCAR-trained and control battalions with respect to baseline characteristics and deployment experiences. The full results of these comparisons are displayed in Table D.2 in Appendix D. The Marines in OSCAR-trained battalions differed significantly at baseline from those in the control battalions in several important ways, such as age, lifetime trauma history, social resources used and recommended to fellow Marines for help with stress, and deployment experiences. In addition, group differences approached but did not attain statistical significance (i.e., $0.05 < p < 0.10$) on rank, parental status, and combat experiences.

The most striking difference between the Marines in OSCAR-trained and control battalions pertains to the types of battalions from which they were sampled: The vast majority of Marines in the OSCAR-trained battalions (89 percent) were in infantry battalions, whereas none of the Marines in control battalions were; all control battalions were service support. However, Marines in OSCAR-trained battalions were not significantly more likely to have been previously deployed than Marines in the control battalions. Given that such characteristics as younger age, trauma history, and deployment experiences have all been shown to increase risk of mental health problems such as PTSD and depression (Brewin, Andrews, and Valentine, 2000; Ozer et al., 2003; Schell and Marshall, 2008), their confounding with the intervention (i.e., OSCAR versus control) necessitated statistical adjustments for these characteristics and experiences.

Climate of Stress Response and Recovery at Baseline

Marines in both the OSCAR-trained and control battalions reported high levels of stress-related trainings in the T1 survey (see Table 3.2). Specifically, 84 percent of Marines in the OSCAR-trained group and 97 percent of Marines in the control group reported one or more prior stress-related trainings, and more than 60 percent of the control group had received four or more stress-related trainings. This attests to the deep penetration of stress-related concerns within the Marine Corps and the familiarity that all Marines are likely to have with basic concepts of stress response. This is particularly important for comparing the OSCAR-trained and control Marines because the control Marines are far from naïve with respect to basic concepts of stress and stress response and official expectations regarding their response to other Marines in distress. The comparison between the Marines in the OSCAR-trained and control battalions, which is the primary focus of this evaluation component, reflects the incremental contribution of OSCAR over and above the stress-related training that all Marines receive.

In addition, healthy stress-related attitudes and the use of positive resources to deal with stress were commonly endorsed in both the OSCAR-trained and control battalions in the T1 survey. At baseline, Marines in both the OSCAR-trained and control groups reported positive expectancies regarding stress response and recovery. Moreover, roughly three-quarters of Marines in each group reported having turned to a fellow Marine for help dealing with stress, and roughly half of Marines in each group reported having turned to a leader for help with stress. However, despite these positive indicators of stress-related attitudes and behaviors, Marines' perceptions of support for help-seeking within their units are moderate in magnitude.

OSCAR's Impact on Stress Response, Help-Seeking Behavior, and Health

Findings on OSCAR's impact on outcomes are organized into three sections: perceptions of stress response and support at the unit level, help-seeking behavior, and health outcomes.

For each outcome, we report the model-adjusted percentages of Marines in the control and OSCAR-trained battalions who showed improvement from pre- to postdeployment on the outcome, defined as movement of any magnitude in a more positive or healthier direction. All analyses were adjusted for differences between Marines in the control and OSCAR-trained battalions on baseline characteristics, including baseline levels of the outcome, and deployment experiences.[9] We also report the estimated treatment effect (i.e., the difference in these percentages between the control and OSCAR-trained battalions).

Perceptions of Stress Response and Support at the Unit Level

As shown in Table 3.3, there were no significant differences between Marines in OSCAR-trained and control battalions in their expectancies regarding stress response and recovery, perceived support for help-seeking, or perceptions of unit support. Thus, contrary to expectation, OSCAR did not appear to have affected perceptions of stress response and support in these domains. However, baseline scores for the whole sample on the measure of expectancies regarding stress response and recovery were already very positive (M = 4.0; SE = 0.01), which left little room for improvement between the T1 and T2 surveys.

Support-Seeking Behavior

We found significant effects of OSCAR on seeking support for one's own stress problems from different types of resources at the unit level. As displayed in Table 3.4, relative to Marines in control battalions, significantly higher proportions of Marines in OSCAR-trained battalions reported having sought support for their own stress problems from fellow Marines, leaders, corpsmen, and any type of resource (fellow Marine, leader, chaplain, corpsman, or unit medical officer) in the T2 survey, even after controlling for group differences in baseline character-

Table 3.3
Comparison of OSCAR-Trained Battalions and Control Battalions on Stress-Related Attitudes, Perceived Support for Stress Response, and Unit Support

Support Domain	Percentage with Improved Perception of Support at T1 Compared with T2 (%)		Estimated Treatment Effect (%)	95% Confidence Interval (%)	p-Value
	Control Battalions (n = 468)	OSCAR-Trained Battalions (n = 839)			
Expectancies regarding stress response and recovery	52	51	−1	−8.3–6.1	0.861
Perceived support for help-seeking	42	44	2	−5.6–9.3	0.648
Unit support	36	40	5[a]	−1.7–10.9	0.367

NOTE: The percentages, estimated treatment effects, and p-values for tests of significance are based on multivariate regression models that adjusted for baseline characteristics and deployment experiences. N = 1,307.

[a] Because of rounding error, the estimated treatment effect does not appear to be equal to the difference between the corresponding point estimates for the control and OSCAR-trained battalions.

---

[9]   Comparisons of Marines in OSCAR-trained and control battalions on postdeployment outcomes that adjust for clustering of Marines within battalions but make no other statistical adjustments (i.e., imputation of missing data, controlling for other variables, propensity score weighting) are available in Table D.3 in Appendix D.

Table 3.4
Comparison of OSCAR-Trained Battalions and Control Battalions on Support-Seeking

Resource	Proportion Using Resource at T2 (%)		Estimated Treatment Effect (%)	95% Confidence Interval (%)	p-Value
	Control Battalions	OSCAR-Trained Battalions			
Used for self					
Fellow Marine*	63	72	10[a]	1.7–18.7	0.000
Leader*	36	43	7	−0.34–14.9	0.006
Corpsman*	23	31	8	1.6–14.9	0.029
Chaplain	20	17	−3	−8.0–3.1	0.057
Unit medical officer	13	11	−2	−6.5–3.1	0.369
Any resource*	72	80	8	−0.7–16.8	0.002
Recommended to peer					
Fellow Marine*	77	86	8[a]	1.2–15.2	0.000
Leader*	51	63	12	4.7–20.3	0.000
Corpsman*	36	51	15	8.2–22.9	0.000
Chaplain	56	53	−3	−9.8–4.3	0.107
Unit medical officer	28	27	−1	−8.3–5.2	0.760
Any resource*	85	90	5	−0.62–10.9	0.000

NOTE: *Any resource* refers to the use of a fellow Marine, leader, chaplain, corpsman, or unit medical officer for support with one's own stress problems or recommending one or more of these types of resources to a fellow Marine for help with his or her (the Marine's) stress problems. All percentages reported in the table are recycled predictions based on adjusted multivariate regression models that control for baseline characteristics and deployment experiences in an effort to isolate the unique contribution of the treatment effect on outcomes.

[a] Because of rounding error, the estimated treatment effect does not appear to be equal to the difference between the corresponding point estimates for the control and OSCAR-trained battalions.

* $p < 0.05$.

istics, including support-seeking behavior, and deployment experiences. Group differences in seeking help from corpsmen might reflect the greater availability of corpsmen in infantry units, which represent the majority of units in the OSCAR-trained group, relative to service-support units, which constitute the entire control group. However, this explanation does not apply to the other sources of informal support that were more commonly used in the OSCAR-trained battalions, including fellow Marines and leaders.

We observed a similar pattern of effects when examining OSCAR's effects on respondents' reports of having recommended various types of resources to fellow Marines for support with stress problems. Relative to Marines in control battalions, significantly higher proportions of Marines in OSCAR-trained battalions reported having recommended to their fellow Marines the use of peers, leaders, corpsmen, and any type of resource (fellow Marine, leader, chaplain, corpsman, or unit medical officer) for help dealing with stress.

It is important to consider a potential alternative explanation for these findings. Members of the OSCAR-trained battalions might have been more likely to seek support because they had greater need for help, resulting from their more-stressful deployment experiences, not because of the OSCAR program. Although this explanation cannot be entirely ruled out, our models include multiple measures of need for support that allow us to control for differences in exposure to stressful experiences during deployment and people's immediate responses to the most stressful experiences they had during deployment. It is also notable that we did not find a difference between the OSCAR-trained and control battalions in the use of medical officers for help, so the observed differences occurred in the specific types of support that are primarily targeted by OSCAR training.

Health Outcomes

Estimates of OSCAR's effects on longer-term health and health behavior outcomes are shown in Table 3.5. None of the differences between the OSCAR-trained and control battalions reaches statistical significance; Marines in the OSCAR-trained battalions did not differ significantly from their peers in control battalions on change in current stress levels, current (past-month) mental health status, high-risk drinking, general health, or occupational impairment. In fact, most of the point estimates are positive, indicating worse outcomes attributable to the OSCAR program, although none of these reaches statistical significance. The corresponding CIs suggest that even a small positive effect of OSCAR on these outcomes is unlikely.

Variation in Outcomes Across OSCAR-Trained Battalions

In addition to examining OSCAR's effects on key outcomes, we examined variation in outcomes by battalion among only the OSCAR-trained battalions. This analysis was intended to illuminate possible variation in the implementation of OSCAR across battalions, as evidence of variation in outcomes by battalion would be consistent with the notion of cross-battalion

Table 3.5
Comparison of OSCAR-Trained and Control Battalions on Health Outcomes

Outcome	Proportion with Outcome at T2 (%)		Estimated Treatment Effect (%)	95% Confidence Interval (%)	p-Value
	Control Battalions	OSCAR-Trained Battalions			
Yellow, orange, or red stress zone	59	60	1	−5.8–8.3	0.845
Probable PTSD	21	25	4	−2.0–11.3	0.132
Probable MDD	19	24	5	−0.29–11.7	0.097
High-risk drinking	27	27	0.58	−6.0–8.2	0.868
General health	16	20	3[a]	−2.3–8.8	0.313
Occupational impairment	36	33	−2[a]	−8.8–3.6	0.415

NOTE: All percentages reported in the table are recycled predictions based on adjusted multivariate regression models that control for baseline characteristics and deployment experiences in an effort to isolate the unique contribution of the treatment effect on outcomes. None of the differences reported in this table attained statistical significance (i.e., all p-values > 0.05).

[a] Because of rounding error, the estimated treatment effect does not appear to be equal to the difference between the corresponding point estimates for the control and OSCAR-trained battalions.

variation in the implementation of OSCAR. To this end, we estimated a series of multivariate regression models in which each outcome was regressed on battalion[10] while adjusting for other baseline characteristics and deployment experiences only among Marines in OSCAR-trained battalions. We found significant differences across the OSCAR-trained battalions in changes over time on all of the outcomes examined (range of Wald chi-square values for omnibus tests of battalion effects: 19.7–2,074.6; all p-values 0.0006 or less), providing support for the hypothesis that the implementation of OSCAR might have varied among battalions. We note, however, that there might be other reasons that outcomes varied across battalions.

Sensitivity Analyses
Multiple Imputation of Missing Data
To understand the extent to which the results of analyses might have been biased by the exclusion of cases with missing data, we estimated a series of multivariate models with multiple imputation of missing data, as described in Appendix C. We found that the pattern of results, i.e., the magnitude and direction of parameter estimates and tests of significance, was nearly identical across the models with and without missing data imputed.[11] The results from models estimated with and without multiple imputation of missing data are juxtaposed in Table E.1 in Appendix E.

Disentangling OSCAR's Effects from Battalion Type
Receipt of OSCAR training was highly confounded with battalion type (infantry versus service support), such that most OSCAR-trained battalions were infantry and all non–OSCAR-trained battalions were service support. In an attempt to disentangle the effect of receipt of OSCAR training from that of battalion type, we estimated multivariate models for the six help-seeking outcomes on which OSCAR had a significant effect in the entire sample within the subset of service-support battalions. We found that the direction of effects was the same for both groups on all six outcomes, and the magnitude of OSCAR's effects on the six outcomes in service-support battalions closely resembled the magnitude of effects obtained within the full sample. These findings indicate that OSCAR's effects described above are more likely attributable to receipt of OSCAR training than to membership in an infantry battalion (as opposed to a service-support battalion). Results from both sets of models are juxtaposed in Table E.2 in Appendix E.

It is useful to consider the impact that the imbalance in battalion type between the OSCAR-trained and control battalions is most likely to have had on the results, even with statistical adjustment for robust measures of deployment experiences. The most likely scenario is that the combat battalions had more-stressful experiences than the noncombat battalions and that this difference was not fully captured in the measures of deployment experience. If this were the case, our models would incompletely adjust for differences in exposures to stress. As a consequence, our estimates of the impact of OSCAR on support-seeking would be overestimates, i.e., attributable to a greater need for help, while the impact of OSCAR on mental

---

[10] Battalion was modeled as a fixed effect represented by a set of dummy-coded indicators, with a battalion that was known to have received OSCAR training with high fidelity to the training guidelines serving as the reference group. Significance of the battalion effect was assessed by the multiple-degree-of-freedom, omnibus test of significance of all dummy-coded indicators.

[11] The results presented in this chapter are from models estimated without imputation of missing data.

health outcomes would be underestimated, i.e., biased toward showing a more negative impact than the program actually had.

Conclusions

Of the short-term outcomes that were the primary targets of OSCAR, we observed significant effects of OSCAR on seeking support for one's own stress problems from peers and leaders, seeking help from corpsmen, and recommending to fellow Marines that they seek support or help for their stress problems from these same resources. OSCAR did not significantly affect any of the other short-term outcomes. Given that expectancies regarding stress response and recovery were already very positive at the outset of the study, the lack of observable attitudinal change between the T1 and T2 surveys is not surprising.

We did not detect any statistically significant effects of OSCAR on the long-term outcomes. In fact, OSCAR's effects on some mental health outcomes were in the opposite direction than that expected; however, these differences were not statistically significant after adjustment for the level of exposure to traumatic events and other deployment-related stressors. These non-significant findings might also not be surprising given that, for many Marines, the T2 survey was administered within just a few months of redeployment. It might be the case that OSCAR has an impact on health outcomes that occur six months, a year, or longer after deployment; however, we were not able to observe this.

Although the observed effects of OSCAR on support- and help-seeking behavior might be viewed as a success of the program, this enthusiasm must be tempered by the lack of clarity regarding the types of assistance and support received by Marines who seek help from one of the unit resources (e.g., peers, leaders, chaplains, corpsmen, or unit medical officers). We can conclude only that OSCAR is connecting more stress-affected Marines to potential sources of assistance without knowing whether these Marines actually receive assistance and, if they do, whether it is appropriate to resolve their stress problems.

The findings from this component of the OSCAR evaluation generalize primarily to lower-ranked, unmarried, childless, active-duty Marines in their early 20s without a history of previous combat deployments. This is the demographic that is at greater risk for mental health problems and thus in greater need of programs that, like OSCAR, are designed to enhance combat and operational stress control. Thus, our findings appropriately generalize to the population that makes up the primary beneficiaries of OSCAR.

Limitations

Despite our efforts to create matched intervention and control groups for this evaluation, the OSCAR-trained and control battalions differed on baseline characteristics and deployment experiences associated with increased risk of mental health problems. These differences are attributable to nonrandom selection of units to receive OSCAR training. Specifically, infantry units, which experience greater combat exposure than service-support units, were prioritized by Marine Corps leadership for receipt of OSCAR training over other types of units. As a result, nearly all of the OSCAR-trained battalions in this evaluation are infantry units, and all of the control battalions are service-support units.

In an effort to correct for the confounding of baseline characteristics and deployment experiences with receipt of OSCAR training, we employed stringent statistical adjustments (i.e., a doubly robust method that incorporated both propensity score weights and covariates in analyses) to control for existing differences between the OSCAR-trained and control battalions. In addition, we conducted a sensitivity analysis designed to disentangle OSCAR's effects from those of battalion type by examining OSCAR's effects within the subset of service-support battalions. For all of the outcomes on which OSCAR exerted a significant effect in the entire sample, the magnitude and direction of OSCAR's effects were similar in the full sample and the subset of service-support battalions.

These statistical adjustments and sensitivity analyses increase confidence in (but do not permit unambiguous attribution of) observed differences between the OSCAR-trained and control groups to OSCAR training. Thus, it is possible that the observed effects of OSCAR on support-seeking and help-seeking behavior are better attributed to other baseline characteristics or deployment experiences whose confounding effects were not effectively eliminated by our statistical adjustments (i.e., residual confounding) or to some other cause not measured in this analysis. Indeed, given the possibility of residual confounding of battalion type with receipt of OSCAR training, it is possible that the differences between OSCAR-trained and control groups reflect differences in need for help with stress or mental health problems resulting from greater combat exposure in the OSCAR-trained battalions, most of which were infantry, relative to the control battalions, all of which were service support.

Another limitation concerns the interpretive ambiguity surrounding the lack of significant effects of OSCAR on long-term outcomes. First, detection of these effects might have been impeded by the methodological limitations of the individual Marine survey—namely, limited precision to detect significant effects due to multiple statistical adjustments for confounds and clustering of observations within battalions. In addition, comparison of the OSCAR-trained battalions with a "stress-training-as-usual" control group, i.e., non–OSCAR-trained battalions in which the majority of participants reported having attended at least one stress-control training class prior to deployment, might have diluted OSCAR's effects to the extent that the other types of stress-control training featured concepts and principles similar to those imparted in OSCAR training. It is also possible that OSCAR in its current form simply does not affect long-term outcomes as intended; that is, the principles and practices for combat stress–management advocated in OSCAR, even if implemented consistently and with fidelity to the program's design, might not be effective tools for improving stress-related attitudes or mental health outcomes. Finally, the lack of significant effects of OSCAR on long-term outcomes might also be attributable to variability in the implementation of OSCAR across battalions. We did not systematically collect information regarding the fidelity of OSCAR's implementation within each of the OSCAR-trained battalions. We know that battalions in the OSCAR-trained condition received OSCAR training in some form, but we do not know how closely the OSCAR training provided to the unit adhered to the OSCAR training guidance. Thus, it is possible that our ability to detect effects of OSCAR was limited by variation in the implementation of OSCAR across battalions. Indeed, consistent with the notion of cross-battalion variation in the implementation of OSCAR, we found significant differences across the OSCAR-trained battalions in changes over time on all of the outcomes examined. However, this is only one possible interpretation of these differences, which might be attributable to other causes.

Summary

In summary, our findings suggest the following:

- Marines in both the control and OSCAR-trained battalions frequently attended stress-control training classes prior to deployment.
- Most Marines had positive expectancies regarding stress response and recovery both before and after deployment.
- Seeking help from informal sources, such as peers, was common.
- Perceptions of support for help-seeking were moderate in magnitude, indicating that perceived stigmatization of help-seeking persists.
- OSCAR increased Marines' use of peers, leaders, and corpsmen for help with stress problems and Marines' recommendations of these same resources to fellow Marines for help with their stress problems.
- OSCAR did not have an effect on expectancies of stress response and recovery, perceived support for help-seeking, or health outcomes.

CHAPTER FOUR

OSCAR Team Members' Perceptions of OSCAR's Impact on Combat and Operational Stress Control: OSCAR Team Member Survey

Deployment presents many opportunities for OSCAR team members to implement the principles and practices of combat stress management conveyed in OSCAR training and to observe how OSCAR affects combat stress management within the unit. As noted previously, the OSCAR team members are typically small-unit leaders who are close to the front lines, know their Marines well, and have the earliest opportunity to recognize and manage the stress problems of Marines in their units. Understanding their perspectives on the climate of stress response and recovery and OSCAR's impact on this climate is essential to gauging the extent to which OSCAR meets the needs of the leaders who have primary responsibility for implementing its principles and practices.

To advance our understanding of OSCAR's currency with OSCAR team members, we designed and fielded a longitudinal survey administered to OSCAR team members.[1] OSCAR team members completed the survey once upon the conclusion of the predeployment OSCAR training (T1) and once after deployment (T2). The OSCAR team member survey assessed perceptions of OSCAR's impact on unit functioning, leadership's ability to manage combat and operational stress problems within the unit, and overall combat and operational stress control from the perspectives of the OSCAR team members who attended predeployment OSCAR training. The survey also assessed perceptions of the climate of stress response and recovery and the frequency of consults, referrals, and requests for assistance received by OSCAR team members for different types of stress problems.

This chapter describes the methods and results of the OSCAR team member survey and discusses its implications for the effectiveness of OSCAR and limitations.

Methods

Sampling and Procedure

Participants for the team member survey were sampled from the same six OSCAR-trained battalions sampled for the individual Marine survey component of the OSCAR evaluation; the sampling of battalions for the individual Marine survey is described in greater detail in Chapter Three and Appendix C. All unit leaders, corpsmen, and chaplains who attended their

---

[1] Although there were some OSCAR extenders who attended the OSCAR training and completed the survey described here, we refer to survey participants as OSCAR team members for simplicity and because the vast majority of survey participants were OSCAR team members (94.4 percent).

units' predeployment OSCAR training and deployed to Iraq or Afghanistan with their units were eligible to participate in the team member survey.[2]

Out of a total of 223 OSCAR training attendees known to have had the opportunity to participate in the T1 survey, 209 Marines chose to participate and 14 Marines declined to participate. However, three of the Marines who completed the T1 survey were later found to be ineligible because they did not deploy to Iraq or Afghanistan with their units as expected. Thus, 206 eligible Marines completed the T1 survey, resulting in a T1 survey cooperation rate of 93.6 percent (206 ÷ [206 + 14]). Of the 206 T1 survey completers, 101 were available for the T2 survey,[3] and 91 completed the survey, yielding a retention rate of 44.2 percent (91 ÷ 206). An analysis of the effect of attrition on the final sample composition is contained in Appendix F.

The T1 survey was administered by paper and pencil to OSCAR team members in a group setting on base right after the unit's OSCAR training was conducted. The amount of time between the dates of the T1 survey administration and deployment varied across battalions, with an average (mean) of 58.6 days (SD = 39.2 days) between these dates (minimum: 13 days; maximum: 6.5 months).

We aimed to administer the T2 survey to all of the OSCAR team members who had completed the T1 survey in a group setting on base approximately two to three months after redeployment from Iraq or Afghanistan. This length of time was intended to allow enough time to pass after redeployment for team members' perceptions of their deployment experiences to stabilize while still surveying them close enough to redeployment that their deployment experiences would be relatively recent and easily recalled. On average, the T2 OSCAR team member survey was conducted 3.7 months (SD = 3.1 months) after redeployment (minimum days: six; maximum days: 303). Variation in the survey administration time frame was attributable primarily to the scheduling constraints of various units. When a respondent was not present at the on-base T2 survey administration, we mailed the T2 survey to the respondent's home address in an effort to maximize the study retention rate.

On-base survey administrations were conducted by a member of the RAND research team or a COSC representative, chaplain, or religious program specialist (RP) who was not in the unit's chain of command so that prospective respondents would not feel coerced to participate. Prior to the survey administrations, respondents were informed that participation was voluntary and that neither their decisions regarding participation nor their survey responses would be shared with anyone outside the RAND research team. Written informed consent was obtained.

Measures

The main purpose of this survey was to assess team members' perceptions of OSCAR's impact on the outcomes it targets (e.g., unit cohesion, morale, and readiness) and team members' atti-

---

[2] According to the OSCAR training guidelines (U.S. Marine Corps, 2011), roughly 5 percent of the unit's leaders, chaplains, corpsmen, and medical personnel are supposed to receive OSCAR training. The leaders who attend the OSCAR training, also referred to as OSCAR team members, are typically officers and senior NCOs selected by the commanding officers on the basis of the leaders' perceived ability to lead effectively, serve as positive role models, and help and mentor Marines with stress problems.

[3] The other 104 T1 survey completers could not be located for the T2 survey, primarily because they had undergone PCSs or the EAS soon after redeployment.

tudes toward stress response and recovery. Given the absence of existing measures of the constructs of interest, we created items to assess these concepts. The domains represented in the survey, the number of items created to tap each domain, and the scale on which items within a given domain were rated are summarized in Table 4.1.

Statistical Analysis

We computed univariate descriptive statistics for individual survey item ratings at T1 and T2 on the sample of OSCAR team members who completed both the T1 and T2 surveys ($N = 91$) and examined the average amount and statistical significance of intra-individual change from T1 to T2 for all items that correspond to the domains shown above in Table 4.1. The average amount of intra-individual change from T1 to T2 was computed as the mean of T2–T1 difference scores. Given the exploratory nature of these tests, we used an alpha level of 0.05 for individual tests of significance.

Because OSCAR training is delivered at the level of the battalion, we expected that a significant amount of the total variance in outcomes would be attributable to differences between battalions. Accordingly, we adjusted for clustering of observations at the battalion level in the estimation of all standard errors and tests of significance.[4]

Results

Participants

Table 4.2 shows the ranks and positions of the T1 and T2 survey completers. OSCAR team members of rank E4–E6 (40 percent) were most commonly represented in the sample, fol-

Table 4.1
Measures of Team Members' Perceptions of OSCAR

Domain	Number of Items	Scale
Attitudes toward stress response and recovery	12	1 (strongly disagree) to 5 (strongly agree)
Perceptions of collaboration between team members and providers	4	1 (strongly disagree) to 5 (strongly agree)
Frequency of consults and referrals received in past month	11	1 (never) to 5 (quite often)
Predeployment expectations and postdeployment perceptions of OSCAR's impact on		
Unit functioning	9	1 (strongly disagree) to 5 (strongly agree)
Leadership's ability to manage stress in the unit	9	1 (not at all) to 4 (to a great extent)
Prevention, identification, and treatment of stress	3	1 (not at all) to 5 (a lot)
Recommended changes to OSCAR's budget	1	Decreased, eliminated, stayed the same, or increased

---

[4] In total, there were six clusters, which correspond to the six OSCAR-trained battalions in the individual Marine survey described in the "Sampling" section of Chapter Three.

Table 4.2
Ranks and Positions of T1 and T2 Survey Completers at T1

Characteristic	Completers (%)
Rank	
E1–E3	15
E4–E6	40
E7–E9	13
O1–O6	32
Position	
Battalion team member (CO, XO, or SgtMaj)	1
Company team member (CO, XO, or first sergeant)	21
Platoon team member (officer or senior enlisted)	72
Navy health care provider, chaplain, or senior corpsman	6

NOTES: CO = commanding officer. XO = executive officer. SgtMaj = sergeant major. N = 91.

lowed by officers (32 percent), junior enlisted (15 percent), and senior NCOs (13 percent). The majority of participants (72 percent) were platoon commanders. Roughly one-fifth of survey participants were company team members (21 percent). Navy health care providers, chaplains, and senior corpsmen made up 6 percent of the sample, and battalion team members constituted 1 percent of the sample.

Attitudes Toward Stress Response and Recovery

Team members were asked about their views related to three topics targeted by OSCAR training: confidence regarding their ability to respond effectively to combat stress reactions, stigmatizing attitudes toward combat stress reactions, and appreciation of the importance of combat stress reactions. Overall, attitudes in these three areas were quite positive at T1 and, apart from a single item, showed no significant change between T1 and T2.

Team members' confidence in their ability to respond to combat stress reactions was assessed through the six items listed in Table 4.3. These items asked about leaders' knowledge of when a Marine might need help with stress-related problems, how to refer such a Marine to help, and about their level of confidence that they can identify problems as problems arise and make appropriate referrals. At T1, team members' responses indicated high levels of confidence on all six items, with average responses ranging from 3.9 (SE = 0.1) to 4.3 (SE = 0.1). There was no statistically significant change in people's responses between T1 and T2 for any of the items.

OSCAR also attempts to influence the culture of Marines by reinforcing positive attitudes toward combat stress reactions, i.e., that anyone might have an adverse stress reaction and that people who have these reactions can recover and return to their prior levels of functioning. The four items listed in Table 4.4 assessed these attitudes among OSCAR team leaders. Attitudes were very positive at T1, ranging from average scores of 3.9 (SE = 0.0) to 4.3 (SE = 0.1) out of 5, and they remained so at T2, ranging from average scores of 4.1 (SE = 0.1) to 4.3 (SE = 0.1). The change from T1 to T2 was statistically significant for one item; on average, survey partici-

Table 4.3
Team Leaders' Confidence in Responding to Combat Stress Reactions

Item Text	T1 Survey M (SE)	T2 Survey M (SE)	Average Change from T1 to T2	
			M (SE)	95% CI
I know how to manage combat and operational stress in my Marines.	4.1 (0.1)	4.2 (0.1)	0.1 (0.1)	−0.0, 0.3
I am confident that I can identify Marines with combat and operational stress problems.	4.1 (0.1)	4.1 (0.1)	0.0 (0.1)	−0.3, 0.3
I know when to refer a Marine with a combat or operational stress problem for higher-level support.	4.2 (0.1)	4.2 (0.1)	0.0 (0.0)	−0.0, 0.1
I know how to refer a Marine with a combat or operational stress problem for higher-level support.	4.2 (0.1)	4.2 (0.1)	0.0 (0.1)	−0.3, 0.3
I know how to use Combat and Operational Stress First Aid (COSFA).	3.9 (0.1)	3.7 (0.2)	−0.2 (0.2)	−0.7, 0.3
I know which stressors or events may cause a combat or operational stress problem.	4.3 (0.1)	4.2 (0.06)	−0.1 (0.1)	−0.3, 0.2

NOTE: Items were rated on a five-point Likert scale where 1 = strongly disagree and 5 = strongly agree; the composite scale score was computed as the average (mean) of all items. Higher scores indicate more-positive attitudes toward stress response and recovery. Average change is computed as the mean of T2–T1 difference scores, where the range of possible scores is −4 to 4. $N = 91$.

Table 4.4
Team Leaders' View of Stigma Associated with Combat Stress Reactions

Item Text	T1 Survey M (SE)	T2 Survey M (SE)	Average Change from T1 to T2	
			M (SE)	95% CI
I make it okay for Marines in my unit to seek help for combat and operational stress problems.	4.3 (0.1)	4.3 (0.1)	0.0 (0.1)	−0.2, 0.2
Most Marines can recover from a stress injury or illness and do their job as well as before.*	3.9 (0.0)	4.2 (0.1)	0.2 (0.1)	0.0, 0.5
I would return a Marine to full duty if he or she had recovered from a stress injury or illness and demonstrated that he or she could do the job.	4.3 (0.1)	4.2 (0.1)	−0.0 (0.1)	−0.2, 0.1
I would treat Marines who recover from stress injuries or illnesses the same as other Marines.	4.2 (0.1)	4.1 (0.1)	−0.1 (0.1)	−0.4, 0.2

NOTE: Items were rated on a five-point Likert scale where 1 = strongly disagree and 5 = strongly agree; the composite scale score was computed as the average (mean) of all items. Higher scores indicate more-positive attitudes toward stress response and recovery. Average change is computed as the mean of T2–T1 difference scores, where the range of possible scores is −4 to 4. $N = 91$.

* Significant change between baseline and follow-up at $p < 0.05$.

pants' attitudes toward recovery from stress injury or illness became more positive between T1 and T2, increasing an average (mean) of 0.2 points (SE = 0.1).

Finally, the questions in Table 4.5 were asked to assess team members' perceptions of the importance of combat stress reactions to individual and unit functioning. Responses indicated a very high level of awareness of the importance of combat stress reactions at T1 and T2 with no significant differences between the two time points. Average responses ranged from 4.4 (SE = 0.1) to 4.6 (SE = 0.1) out of 5.

Perceptions of Collaboration Between Team Members and Providers

One of the goals of OSCAR is to improve collaborations between operational leaders and mental health providers by embedding mental health providers within forward-deployed units. We asked team members at baseline and at follow-up about their perceptions of these collaborative relationships. As shown in Table 4.6, survey respondents endorsed neutral or slightly positive perceptions of collaboration and communication between team members and providers at

Table 4.5
Team Leaders' Appreciation of the Importance of Combat Stress Reactions

Item Text	T1 Survey M (SE)	T2 Survey M (SE)	Average Change from T1 to T2	
			M (SE)	95% CI
Even the strongest Marine can be affected by a combat or operational stress problem.	4.6 (0.1)	4.5 (0.1)	−0.1 (0.1)	−0.3, 0.1
Combat and operational stress problems that aren't addressed can compromise the mission readiness of my Marines.	4.6 (0.0)	4.4 (0.1)	−0.1 (0.1)	−0.3, 0.0

NOTE: Items were rated on a five-point Likert scale where 1 = strongly disagree and 5 = strongly agree; the composite scale score was computed as the average (mean) of all items. Higher scores indicate more-positive attitudes toward stress response and recovery. Average change is computed as the mean of T2–T1 difference scores, where the range of possible scores is −4 to 4. N = 91.

Table 4.6
Perceptions of Collaboration Between Line Leaders and Providers

Item Text	T1 Survey M (SE)	T2 Survey M (SE)	Average Change from T1 to T2	
			M (SE)	95% CI
Line team members and providers communicate frequently about individual Marines.	3.4 (0.0)	3.6 (0.1)	0.1 (0.1)	−0.2, 0.4
It is easy for providers to talk to line team members about the needs of Marines.	3.4 (0.0)	3.6 (0.1)	0.2 (0.1)	−0.1, 0.4
In my unit, line team members and providers collaborate effectively.	3.4 (0.1)	3.5 (0.1)	0.1 (0.1)	−0.2, 0.4
In my unit, line team members and providers use resources and tools for stress management efficiently.	3.4 (0.1)	3.6 (0.1)	0.2 (0.1)	−0.1, 0.5
Composite scale score (mean of 4 scale items)	3.4 (0.1)	3.6 (0.1)	0.1 (0.1)	−0.1, 0.3

NOTE: Items were rated on a five-point Likert scale where 1 = strongly disagree and 5 = strongly agree; the composite scale score is computed as the average (mean) of all items. Higher scores on individual item ratings and the composite scale score indicate more-positive perceptions of collaboration between team members and providers. Average change is computed as the mean of T2–T1 difference scores, where the range of possible scores is −4 to 4. N = 91.

both time points. Ratings averaged 3.4 (SE = 0.1) at baseline and ranged from 3.5 (SE = 0.1) to 3.6 (SE = 0.1) at follow-up. Although there were small increases in each item in the T2 compared with the T1 survey, none of these reached statistical significance. Similarly, participants' mean scores on all four items did not significantly change between the T1 and T2 assessments.

Types of Consults, Referrals, or Requests for Assistance Received in Role as Team Member or Provider

OSCAR was designed to increase the frequency with which Marines use informal sources of support, OSCAR team members in particular, for combat stress–related problems. To assess whether team members received more consults after being trained, we asked them to indicate how often they had received consults, referrals, or requests for assistance for various types of problems in the past month at T1 and T2 (Table 4.7). In general, team members reported infrequent consults, referrals, or requests for assistance at both time points. The only type of problem for which the frequency of consults increased significantly between T1 and T2 was combat stress. The frequency of consults for peer conflict and spouse or partner conflict decreased significantly between T1 and T2. No other significant differences between T1 and T2 were observed in this domain.

Table 4.7
Average Frequencies of Contacts or Encounters for Different Types of Problems About Which the Team Member Has Been Consulted in the Past Month

Type of Problem	T1 Survey M (SE)	T2 Survey M (SE)	Average Change from T1 to T2	
			M (SE)	95% CI
Stress from combat*	1.8 (0.2)	2.2 (0.1)	0.5 (0.2)	0.0, 0.9
Stress from military operations other than combat	2.6 (0.1)	2.5 (0.1)	−0.0 (0.2)	−0.5, 0.4
Financial problems	2.7 (0.2)	2.5 (0.1)	−0.2 (0.1)	−0.6, 0.1
Misconduct or other legal problems	2.7 (0.2)	2.5 (0.1)	−0.2 (0.2)	−0.7, 0.3
Peer conflict*	2.6 (0.1)	2.2 (0.1)	−0.4 (0.1)	−0.5, −0.2
Spouse or partner conflict*	2.7 (0.1)	2.5 (0.1)	−0.1 (0.1)	−0.3, −0.0
Depression	2.0 (0.1)	2.0 (0.1)	−0.1 (0.1)	−0.3, 0.2
Anxiety	2.2 (0.1)	2.0 (0.1)	−0.2 (0.1)	−0.4, 0.1
Substance use	2.1 (0.1)	2.0 (0.1)	−0.1 (0.2)	−0.7, 0.5
Suicidal thoughts	1.6 (0.1)	1.7 (0.1)	0.1 (0.1)	−0.2, 0.3
Other	1.5 (0.3)	1.9 (0.3)	0.6 (0.2)	−0.1, 1.2

NOTE: Items were rated on a five-point scale where 1 = never and 5 = quite often. Higher scores on individual scale items indicate greater frequency of having received consults for a particular type of problem. Average change is computed as the mean of T2–T1 difference scores, where the range of possible scores is –4 to 4. Average change scores greater than 0 and less than or equal to 4 indicate increases in the frequency of consults from T1 to T2. Average change scores less than 0 and greater than or equal to –4 indicate decreases in the frequency of consults from T1 to T2. N = 91.

* Significant change between baseline and follow-up at $p < 0.05$.

Predeployment Expectations Versus Postdeployment Perceptions of the Beneficial Effects of OSCAR

Because OSCAR team members are integral to the success of OSCAR, their attitudes toward the program and its impact on key target outcomes were assessed at baseline and follow-up. At T1, we asked team members about their expectations of the program. At T2, we asked them about their perceptions of how OSCAR affected the same outcomes during their most recent deployments. Expectations and perceptions of OSCAR were assessed for three domains: unit functioning and readiness; leadership's ability to manage stress in their units; and stress prevention, identification, and treatment.

Unit Functioning and Readiness

As shown in Table 4.8, on average, respondents' expectations and perceptions of OSCAR's impact on nearly all aspects of unit functioning before and after deployment were neutral or slightly positive about OSCAR's benefits on unit functioning. The items that received the highest ratings at T1 and T2, indicating that OSCAR most benefited these areas, were the readiness of individual Marines and the mission readiness of the respondent's unit as a whole.

Table 4.8
Expectations and Perceptions of OSCAR's Impact on Unit Cohesion, Readiness, and Morale

Item Text	Predeployment Expectations M (SE)	Postdeployment Perceptions M (SE)	Average Difference Between Expectations and Perceptions M (SE)	95% CI
OSCAR has improved the confidence of Marines in my unit.*	3.6 (0.2)	3.2 (0.1)	−0.4 (0.1)	−0.8, −0.0
OSCAR has increased the commitment of Marines in my unit.*	3.4 (0.1)	3.1 (0.1)	−0.4 (0.1)	−0.6, −0.1
OSCAR has enhanced the readiness of individual Marines.	3.8 (0.1)	3.4 (0.1)	−0.4 (0.2)	−0.9, 0.0
OSCAR has improved the mission readiness of my unit as a whole.*	3.8 (0.1)	3.4 (0.1)	−0.4 (0.1)	−0.7, −0.2
OSCAR has improved cohesion in my unit.*	3.5 (0.1)	3.1 (0.1)	−0.5 (0.1)	−0.7, −0.2
OSCAR has improved morale in my unit.*	3.5 (0.1)	3.1 (0.1)	−0.4 (0.1)	−0.7, −0.2
OSCAR has increased the productivity of Marines in my unit.*	3.5 (0.1)	3.0 (0.1)	−0.5 (0.1)	−0.6, −0.3
OSCAR has decreased the number of sick call days in my unit.*	3.0 (0.07)	2.7 (0.1)	−0.3 (0.1)	−0.6, −0.1
OSCAR has decreased stigma about stress problems.*	3.6 (0.17)	3.2 (0.2)	−0.4 (0.0)	−0.5, −0.3

NOTE: All items in the table above reflect the wording used in the T2 survey to assess postdeployment perceptions of OSCAR's impact; the words "OSCAR has . . . " were replaced with the words "OSCAR will . . . " to assess predeployment expectations in the T1 survey. Higher item ratings indicate more-positive expectations and perceptions of OSCAR's impacts. Average intra-individual discrepancies between predeployment expectations and postdeployment perceptions are computed as the mean of difference scores created by subtracting ratings of items assessing predeployment expectations from ratings of the items assessing the corresponding postdeployment perceptions. Items in the table were rated on a five-point Likert scale where 1 = strongly disagree and 5 = strongly agree. The range of possible scores for mean discrepancies between predeployment expectations and postdeployment perceptions is −4 to 4. $N = 91$.

* Significant change between baseline and follow-up at $p < 0.05$.

In general, predeployment expectations for OSCAR's impact received higher ratings than post-deployment perceptions of how OSCAR actually affected unit functioning.

Leadership's Ability to Manage Stress in the Unit

As Table 4.9 shows, most respondents endorsed modest expectations and perceptions of OSCAR's impact on leaders' ability to manage operational stress in the unit before and after deployment. The items that received the highest ratings at T1 and T2, indicating that OSCAR

Table 4.9
Expectations and Perceptions of OSCAR's Impacts on Unit Leadership's Ability to Manage Combat and Operational Stress Problems in Their Units

Item Text	Predeployment Expectations M (SE)	Postdeployment Perceptions M (SE)	Average Difference Between Expectations and Perceptions	
			M (SE)	95% CI
OSCAR has enhanced the ability of leadership to conduct training to develop physical, tactical, and mental strength and endurance among Marines.*	2.9 (0.1)	2.5 (0.1)	−0.4 (0.1)	−0.7, −0.2
OSCAR has enhanced the ability of leadership to maintain cohesion within the unit.*	2.9 (0.1)	2.5 (0.1)	−0.4 (0.1)	−0.7, −0.1
OSCAR has enhanced the ability of leadership to maintain the esprit de corps of the unit.*	2.7 (0.1)	2.4 (0.1)	−0.3 (0.1)	−0.5, −0.2
OSCAR has enhanced the ability of leadership to monitor the stress zones of Marines.	3.2 (0.2)	2.8 (0.1)	−0.4 (0.2)	−0.8, 0.0
OSCAR has enhanced the ability of leadership to help Marines manage their own stress.*	3.2 (0.1)	2.6 (0.1)	−0.6 (0.2)	−1.0, −0.2
OSCAR has enhanced the ability of leadership to ensure adequate rest and recovery.*	2.7 (0.1)	2.3 (0.1)	−0.4 (0.1)	−0.7, −0.1
OSCAR has enhanced the ability of leadership to access the appropriate level of care for Marines with stress problems.*	3.2 (0.1)	2.8 (0.1)	−0.4 (0.1)	−0.6, −0.2
OSCAR has enhanced the ability of leadership to reduce stigma related to talking about and receiving help for stress problems within the unit.*	3.0 (0.1)	2.7 (0.1)	−0.3 (0.1)	−0.5, −0.1
OSCAR has enhanced the ability of leadership to reintegrate Marines with stress injuries or illnesses back into the unit.*	3.0 (0.1)	2.6 (0.1)	−0.4 (0.1)	−0.6, −0.2

NOTE: All items in the table above reflect the wording used in the T2 survey to assess postdeployment perceptions of OSCAR's impact; the words "OSCAR has . . . " were replaced with the words "OSCAR will . . . " to assess predeployment expectations in the T1 survey. Higher item ratings indicate more-positive expectations and perceptions of OSCAR's impacts. Average intra-individual discrepancies between predeployment expectations and postdeployment perceptions are computed as the mean of difference scores created by subtracting ratings of items assessing predeployment expectations from ratings of the items assessing the corresponding postdeployment perceptions. Items in this table were rated on a four-point Likert scale where 1 = not at all and 4 = to a great extent. The range of possible scores for mean discrepancies between predeployment expectations and postdeployment perceptions is −3 to 3. $N = 91$.

* Significant change between baseline and follow-up at $p < 0.05$.

seemed most relevant to these areas, were leaders' abilities to monitor the stress zones of Marines and access the appropriate level of care. On average, predeployment expectations for OSCAR's impact on leadership's ability received higher ratings than postdeployment perceptions of how OSCAR actually affected leadership's ability.

Stress Prevention, Identification, and Treatment

As shown in Table 4.10, team members expected that OSCAR would improve the prevention, identification, and treatment of stress problems moderately or quite a bit. After returning from deployment, respondents tended to report that OSCAR had improved the prevention, identification, and treatment of stress problems only a little or moderately. On average, respondents' ratings of expectations and perceptions of OSCAR's impact on stress prevention, identification, and treatment decreased by 0.6 (SE = 0.2), 0.6 (SE = 0.2), and 0.7 (SE = 0.2), respectively, between T1 and T2.

Recommendations for Changes to the Budget for OSCAR

When we asked respondents whether, if it were up to them, the budget for OSCAR would be increased, decreased, eliminated, or would stay the same,[5] the majority indicated that they

Table 4.10
Expectations and Perceptions of OSCAR's Impacts on the Management of Combat and Operational Stress Problems

Item Text	Predeployment Expectations M (SE)	Postdeployment Perceptions M (SE)	Average Difference Between Expectations and Perceptions	
			M (SE)	95% CI
OSCAR has improved prevention of combat and operational stress problems*	3.3 (0.2)	2.6 (0.1)	−0.6 (0.2)	−1.1, −0.1
OSCAR has improved identification of Marines with combat and operational stress problems.*	3.5 (0.2)	3.0 (0.1)	−0.6 (0.2)	−1.0, −0.1
OSCAR has improved treatment of combat and operational stress problems at the unit level.*	3.5 (0.2)	2.8 (0.1)	−0.7 (0.2)	−1.3, −0.2

NOTE: All items in the table above reflect the wording used in the T2 survey to assess postdeployment perceptions of OSCAR's impact; the words "OSCAR has . . . " were replaced with the words "OSCAR will . . . " to assess predeployment expectations in the T1 survey. Higher item ratings indicate more-positive expectations and perceptions of OSCAR's impacts. Average intra-individual discrepancies between predeployment expectations and postdeployment perceptions are computed as the mean of difference scores created by subtracting ratings of items assessing predeployment expectations from ratings of the items assessing the corresponding postdeployment perceptions. Items in this section were rated on a five-point Likert scale where 1 = not at all and 5 = a lot. The range of possible scores for mean discrepancies between predeployment expectations and postdeployment perceptions is −4 to 4. $N = 91$.

* Significant change between baseline and follow-up at $p < 0.05$.

---

[5] The actual survey question was as follows: "If it were up to me, the budget for the OSCAR program would be . . . ." Response options included *eliminated*, *decreased*, *stay the same*, or *increased*.

would increase the budget (T1: 30 percent, n = 55; T2: 8 percent, n = 7) or have it stay the same (T1: 52 percent, n = 96; T2: 64 percent, n = 56) at both time points. Relatively small proportions of respondents expressed a preference for the budget to be decreased (T1: 6 percent, n = 33; T2: 13 percent, n = 11) or eliminated (T1: 12 percent, n = 22; T2: 15 percent, n = 13).

Conclusions

Consistent with findings from the individual Marine survey, findings from the OSCAR team member survey indicated widespread positive attitudes toward stress response and recovery both before and after deployment. OSCAR team members' perceptions of communication and collaboration between line leaders and providers regarding stress problems in the unit, although less positive than attitudes toward stress response and recovery, were generally neutral or positive. These findings reinforce the notion that the climate of stress response and recovery in the Marine Corps is generally positive.

OSCAR team members reported that they seldom received consults, referrals, or requests for assistance during the past month in both the T1 and T2 surveys. One interpretation of these findings is that survey participants were in units in which stress problems were relatively uncommon, which would have limited opportunities for consultations and requests for assistance with stress problems. Alternatively, it might be that stress problems were common and that OSCAR team members were seldom asked to provide consultation or other forms of assistance for stress problems for reasons that are unclear. Assuming the latter, one reason that OSCAR team members might have been infrequently consulted is that Marines in the unit were unaware of who the OSCAR team members in their units were and so did not fully appreciate or draw on them as resources for help with stress. Alternatively, Marines who were experiencing stress problems might have preferred to seek help from someone, such as a trusted peer or a leader who was a "natural mentor," rather than an OSCAR team member who was less well-known to them.

Other possible explanations for the infrequency of stress consultations pertain to the timing of the survey and the wording of the question. The time frame of the past month might not have covered stressful periods during deployment when consults, referrals, and requests for assistance might have been more frequent; for example, the postdeployment survey was often administered soon after the unit's return from block leave, which might have limited occasion for such consults or other requests for help to be made. Second, because OSCAR team members are intended to serve as informal sources of support to Marines in their units, it might be that their consultations and requests for assistance with stress problems are so informally received, i.e., are broached in the course of casual conversation, that team members might not have considered them "consultations," which is a more formal term.

Team members' perceptions of OSCAR's impact on a wide array of areas relevant to combat and operational stress control indicated modest enthusiasm for OSCAR's impacts both before deployment (right after OSCAR training) and after deployment. On nearly all of the domains assessed, postdeployment perceptions of OSCAR's impact were consistently less positive than predeployment expectations. These differences might simply reflect that enthusiasm for OSCAR is likely to be greatest right after the training, when the positive messages conveyed in the OSCAR training are easily recalled and very salient to OSCAR team members. After several months have passed since attending the training, OSCAR team members might have greater difficulty recalling the principles of OSCAR and thus might be less inclined to endorse positive perceptions of its impact. Alternatively, it might be that, immediately after OSCAR training and prior to deployment, OSCAR team members understood OSCAR on a more theoretical level, and implementing the principles of OSCAR in real-world situations during deployment might have been more challenging than initially expected. Thus, the practical challenges of applying the principles of OSCAR to actual combat and operational stress problems encountered in theater might have diminished enthusiasm for its benefits. Another possible explanation of these findings is that OSCAR team members were disappointed about having been consulted infrequently regarding stress problems and thus having little opportunity to apply the principles and practices learned in OSCAR training. However, it should be noted that, both before and after deployment, upward of 70 percent of OSCAR team members perceived that the budget for OSCAR should be increased or stay the same. In general, then, it appears that team members consider OSCAR's benefits sufficient to sustain it.

Limitations

In interpreting findings from this survey, a couple of caveats warrant mention. First, the small sample size limited power to detect significant change over time in the attitudes and perceptions assessed in the survey. However, we did detect several significant differences of interest, particularly with respect to predeployment expectations and postdeployment perceptions of OSCAR's impact. Second, we do not have comparison data on the broader population of Marines who have been trained as OSCAR team members to determine how closely our sample of OSCAR team members resembles the broader population. Thus, the extent to which findings from this survey generalize to the broader population of OSCAR team members is unknown.

Summary

In summary, the key findings from the pre- and postdeployment OSCAR team member surveys are as follows:

- Most team members endorsed attitudes toward stress response and recovery that were consistently positive before and after returning from deployment.
- In general, respondents reported that they infrequently received consults for most types of problems both before and after deployment.
- Team members' expectations for OSCAR's impact on unit cohesion, mission readiness, and morale; leadership's ability to manage combat and operational stress problems in their units; and the prevention, identification, and management of combat stress problems were significantly more positive than their postdeployment perceptions of how OSCAR had actually affected these domains.
- The great majority of respondents indicated that, if it were up to them, they would increase the budget for OSCAR or have it stay the same both before and after deployment.

CHAPTER FIVE

Officers' and Enlisted Marines' Perspectives on OSCAR: Focus Groups with Marines

In this chapter, we present the methods and findings of focus groups with Marines and discuss the implications of those findings for OSCAR's effects on the climate of stress response and recovery within the Marine Corps.

Methods

Participants in the focus groups included OSCAR-trained team members, as well as some non–OSCAR-trained enlisted Marines who had varying degrees of familiarity with the OSCAR program. Our contacts in the COSC office helped to identify focus group participants. Seven focus groups sampled from five battalions were conducted on base (the composition of each group is shown in Table 5.1). Each of the focus groups included six to 14 Marines. A RAND researcher led the discussions with a set of questions developed to stimulate broad discussion of combat-related stressors, as well as more-detailed discussion about OSCAR. Participants were also asked to provide recommendations for improving the management of combat stress–related problems in the Marine Corps. The focus groups were audio recorded and transcribed, and the transcripts were analyzed using thematic analysis methods.

Table 5.1
Focus Groups Conducted for the OSCAR Evaluation

Group	Number of Participants	Group Composition	OSCAR Training Status
1	14	NCOs	All OSCAR-trained team members
2	7	NCOs and officers	All OSCAR-trained team members
3	6	Enlisted	No OSCAR-trained team members
4	10	Enlisted	Mostly OSCAR-trained team members
5	9	NCOs and officers	Some OSCAR-trained team members
6	10	Enlisted	No OSCAR-trained team members
7	7	Enlisted	No OSCAR-trained team members

Results

This section is organized according to the key themes and subthemes identified. Key themes include variation in views of combat stress programs, recognition that combat stress is a real problem, emphasis on peer relations and effective leadership in effective management of combat stress problems, and valuation of OSCAR as a platform for stress response that aligns well with military culture and routine. Illustrative quotes are provided for each theme.

Participants Voiced Varied Views of Combat Stress–Management Programs
Participants Expressed Some Resistance to Externally Imposed Combat Stress Programs
The Marines who participated in the focus groups expressed complex and sometimes contradictory ideas about the training programs, including OSCAR, that the Marine Corps has put in place to improve the management of combat stress. On the one hand, many of the Marines expressed in strong terms their sense that these systems are imposed from outside and that they conflict with spontaneous relationships among Marines that arise in the course of their work. Externally imposed systems are considered to be ineffectual. As one Marine explained,

> As soon as something that is supposed to be an idea or a feeling of genuine caring becomes regimented, now it's stuck in a block. It's no longer training anymore; it's forced learning . . . . Generally speaking, when you put a rule on something, Marines are going to push that boundary and attempt to break it. Training in the sense of administrative training is looked at really different than warfighter training. The warfighter training becomes muscle memory for Marines. They do it till they can't get it wrong; that's what makes them professional. The administrative side of the house is forced upon; it almost becomes a check in a box.

To an extent, even the relatively discreet methods of the OSCAR program face the same resistance:

> Any flow chart, color system, that really doesn't matter to me; I'm not going to remember that. . . . Bottom line is you just need to talk to the guy, work through the issue; it doesn't matter what the frickin color is. . . . It's so unexact that them trying to put it in a color code is . . . ridiculous.

Participants Perceived That the Amount of Combat Stress–Control Training Received Is Excessive
"Overkill" was used in several of the focus groups to describe the volume of combat stress–management training they received. Many participants agreed with the Marine quoted below in their view that there was *too much* training about combat stress:

> I think one time and you're done. We got hit four, five times before we left and I don't know how many times since we've been back, so it's definitely overkill.

An important point that these quotes also show is that Marines did not systematically differentiate between OSCAR and other programs related to combat stress. To the contrary, all these trainings tended to be grouped together into a single category, along with other psychosocial functioning programs (e.g., sexual harassment programs). For the most part, these are collectively viewed as perhaps necessary but ineffective and externally imposed. Wariness about this general category of program was applied to the OSCAR program as well.

Participants Expressed Concern That Stress-Control Trainings Might Inadvertently Sensitize Marines to Stress

Wariness about combat stress–control training went as far as concern that the training has negative effects on performance and morale by oversensitizing people to potential stress-related problems. This concern arose independently in several focus groups. For instance, Marines are concerned that "stress" is becoming an overused excuse for common disciplinary problems:

> Yeah, when I yell at a Marine for not having his room clean, he's like, "oh I'm stressed out because I didn't do something I was supposed to do." It kind of makes me mad that it's like that now [stress is like an excuse]. But that's how it is, so . . . But people milk it, too.

There was not much doubt among the focus group participants that this results from combat stress–control training and is reinforced by an overarching culture, inside and outside the military, that unduly focuses attention on stress. For example, one participant said,

> When I came to boot camp, the whole "hey I'm stressed out" thing didn't apply. Everyone seemed fine. And now everyone's so stressed. I don't know. I was fine without the whole stress class. I don't know about you guys, but the more they talk about it, the more Marines are like, "yeah I actually am stressed."

> [Moderator] Do you think that's because people are more stressed, or because they're talking about it more?

> Because they're talking about it more. It's almost like a commercial for food. It's like you see a commercial for T-bone steak and you really want it. And like, they offered this class, they show you how people are stressed, then people start thinking, "Wow, I feel like that all the time."

———

> Giving the tools to the leaders and the mentors, and the guys that have a little maturity and can put it into context is good but I almost felt , . . . the young Marines just got bombarded with this operational stress. I think it almost convinced some of them that they had it when they were fine and everyone was like, "Are you okay? Are you okay?" "Well I thought I was, but maybe I'm not. Everyone's telling me that I should be screwed up right now, maybe I am screwed up right now."

Participants Considered Combat Stress to Be a Real Problem

Despite these criticisms of OSCAR and apparent skepticism about the entire concept of a combat stress–response program, the Marines who participated in the focus groups uniformly considered combat stress to be a real and serious concern. Rather than claim that these programs are unnecessary, Marines emphasized that combat stress management has always been an important part of Marine Corps culture. Participants perceived OSCAR to be a set of formal methods for accomplishing goals that have always been accomplished informally:

> I think we've always had something here; whether you call it OSCAR or not, I think we've all taken care of each other around here. . . . We've just never put a name on it or formalized it.

———

> Seemed to be a course for things that we've already been taught to do the whole time I've been in the Marine Corps, small-unit leadership–type stuff, they just put it in a course, basically. We've always looked out for our Marines and been looked out for by our highers and our peers, talk to each other, try to do it, if you do find problems, try to help them out. Something we've informally done since 1775 and now they've put it in a course . . . to put an emphasis on it.

Even without OSCAR, some argued, Marines were already sensitive to the changes in behavior that signaled serious combat stress–related problems:

> Yeah, we have squad leaders and team leaders and stuff like that; usually they work with a little group of Marines. So they would notice more often, even if they're not OSCAR-trained. The team leader would recognize, "Hey, this Marine, he's my Marine; he's acting different." So usually [the squad or team leader] would go up and talk to [the afflicted Marine], even if he didn't have the training, just to see if there's something wrong.

Participants Emphasized Peer Relationships and Effective Leadership

The focus group discussions brought out two important aspects of the informal systems that Marines believe are effective in managing combat stress in practice: strong peer-to-peer relationships and effective leadership. Peers work together intensively, and, whether they want to or not, they come to know one another so well that they are aware when someone's behavior changes because of stress:

> We don't have a problem here in our unit because these guys know each other, they eat, sleep, breathe, do everything with them because they work in very small units, very small teams, and they're brothers. Whether they like each other or they don't like each other, they're brothers, and it's easier for the Marines to pick up the indicators.

Moreover, peers are much easier to approach than a representative of a more formal system of assistance. For example, peers are on the front line when it comes to seeking help for problems:

> Because when you first join the Marine Corps, you're going to be stressed out, as a PFC [private first class] and a Private. . . . You wouldn't want to take it to your chain of command. You're going to want to take it to your peers. And if there's a really big problem, his corporal will come up to us.

Peers can also suggest help when they observe that another is stressed:

> If I had a friend that was seriously suffering from stress from before, I would definitely go up to him and try to help him out, 'cause you're on a level with him. And it's not like someone random coming up and is like, "Hey, what's wrong with you, man?" You know?

These comments are not hard to understand in the highly structured world of the Marine Corps, in which approaching a superior with a problem sets in motion a whole raft of consequences that a young Marine might be unable to understand or predict. A peer, on the other hand, can give informal feedback without being required to report up the chain of command.

Leadership quality came up as a critical factor in stress management in several of the focus groups, with Marines expressing the idea that good leadership skills address combat stress reactions and mitigate their impact, with or without specific training programs, such as OSCAR. Good leadership involves spending time to get to know individual Marines under one's command so that there is trust and a basis for noticing behavioral changes. For instance, one participant reported,

> I think just spending more one-on-one time with them. I don't really think you need anything, you just need to actually be a leader and get involved with your Marines instead of always passing it down to a lower level. You need to actually get more face time with them.

One participant related the following story as evidence that good leadership meant effective combat stress management:

> I would always talk to my Marines, and I got to know them personally so I could tell differences in their performance, and I would talk to them, and I found out one of my guys' twin brother committed suicide. And it pushed up; I got him home to take care of all the affairs, and he came back, and I cut him slack for a couple months. I gave him some space, and he's doing just fine now. But I know other team leaders that don't know their Marines at all; they completely shut them out. It's just, "you're baloney; you do what I say." I know there's a period at the beginning, when you first get your Marines, you gotta put them in their place, but after a couple months, you need to know your Marines, and that's on the small-unit leaders.

The leadership theme is so strong among Marines that even those who were trained in OSCAR tended to think of their own role as OSCAR team members in terms of leadership, rather than in terms of specialized mental health expertise:

> We don't really address it as "hey, we're OSCAR mentors, come to us." It's just part of our leadership role anyway.

The emphasis that Marines put on peer-to-peer relationships and leadership qualities reinforces the impression of a strong resistance against formalizing aspects of interpersonal relationships in the service of managing combat stress and a corresponding tendency to normalize combat stress management as implicit expectations and mutual responsibilities that are informal aspects of relationships among Marines.

Participants Prefer Trainers with Combat Experience and "Natural" Mentors

In keeping with their emphasis on "organic" informal peer-to-peer over "external" clinical support, participants voiced related concerns about the OSCAR training sessions and the designated OSCAR mentors. With respect to the trainings, there was a strong preference for trainers who had combat experience and could therefore speak directly from their experience to the concerns of Marines:

> Maybe if you just had success stories of people using OSCAR . . . Marines [who] actually used OSCAR, who sought help and got integrated back to my unit. If you had more people who actually used it, who had it happen to them and have them speak about it, it would probably hit closer to home than just having [an instructor] speak.

————

> I think, as long as the Marines hear it from people they know, instead of watching it on some video, that will be beneficial.

————

> He's exactly 100 percent right: Someone who's a combat vet, preferably a Marine, someone who was in the infantry—they understand us better than anyone else would have, not to say anything bad about the professionals that do come in, but the bottom line is: If I'm looking at someone who's never been in the military, it's like, "How can you relate?" and you can't—you can't relate. I don't care how many people you deal with, you can understand but you can't relate and completely understand like someone would that's actually been in your situation.

Similar concerns were raised regarding the OSCAR team members (mentors). Marines were resistant to the idea that OSCAR mentors designated as such by their commanders are the best source of support. They prefer to consult with mentors of their own choosing:

> I think that's how the Marine Corps came up with the mentorship . . . but I completely disagree with it. You're not going to assign me a mentor; I'm going to pick my mentor. I can't sit down and talk to this guy if I think he's a shithead.

Mentoring that occurs naturally in the course of duty is thought to be more effective than mentoring occurring as part of a prescribed procedure:

> I'm more like, one-on-one time is riding in the truck together, on the way to the field or getting them their gun while they're in the field. . . .

————

I think that's the best time too because, when I've been counseled—you know, the Lieutenant brings you in—it's been like, "What do you like doing?" and you tell him, and it's sort of like a checklist; he's like, "Okay, that's you! Next." But if you're in the field and he's like, "What do you like doing for sports? What position did you play in high school?" it's more natural; it's more social as opposed to I'm doing this because I have to, I don't care about you; I'm just checking a box to know my Marines.

In fact, focus group participants suggested that designating a person as an OSCAR mentor could actually make it more difficult to seek help from that person:

I think that already, that support already exists; the Marines know that the leaders that they're going to go to . . . have that experience and have knowledge, wisdom, their trust, so they're going to go talk to them anyways, so this is just something to give them more tools, but I think that, if you were to put an OSCAR title in the job description, it would hurt that.

Participants Who Had Received OSCAR Training Appreciate It as a "Platform"

Although the focus group participants emphasized the value of informal, nonspecialized methods for managing combat stress, those with direct experience of the OSCAR program also appreciated the value of OSCAR. As illustrated in the quote below, participants appreciated that OSCAR provided an organizing system, a "platform" in the words of this Marine, for responding to serious problems of combat stress without disrupting military routine:

OSCAR just gave you a more professional kind of period of instruction when dealing with combat stress. I mean, we've all experienced it at some point, even before the OSCAR training, but that just kind of ties everything together, gives it a platform.

Where participants were positive about OSCAR, they emphasized the complementarity between the program and existing informal support networks.

What the OSCAR is supposed to do and what we're supposed to do as leaders is acknowledge that [stress is] occurring and allow the Marines to believe that they have a voice, without retribution. The talk about the stress—it ruins everyone's life; it's not specific to the Marine Corps. It occurs every single day and, with the OSCAR and the combat stress and other programs, we're just acknowledging it.

Another participant commented about OSCAR: "It gives us a common language to talk about stress."

Conclusions

The focus groups provide a window into how Marines evaluate and respond to issues of combat stress and the OSCAR program in particular. The discussions revealed some persistent tensions that have been described in the literature on combat stress for many years and have informed the design of OSCAR. These themes include the inevitability of stress reactions in combat, resistance to clinical intervention in favor of normalizing, a preference for informal supports wherever possible, and a concern that stress reactions and mental health care for stress reactions are highly stigmatized. Recent research also suggests that stigma associated with mental health care is a significant barrier to care, particularly for active-duty troops (Hoge et al., 2004; Kim et al., 2010). Marines in the focus groups favor nonclinical approaches to combat stress, but they do not rule out the occasional need for clinical intervention. Marines are concerned that negative stigma might prevent people from seeking help that would improve readiness, but they are also concerned that an overemphasis on stress response can lead to abuse, overdiagnosis, and dependence, which also adversely affect readiness. This concern with potential overdiagnosis of mental health problems also echoes persistent concerns in the scientific literature (Wessely, 2005).

These concerns closely reflect those of the designers of the OSCAR program, who aimed to design a program that expanded resources to support Marines in combat while minimizing the use of potentially stigmatizing clinical intervention. This is important because the ultimate impact of OSCAR and other combat stress–control training programs depends in part on the extent to which Marines buy into the program's concepts of combat stress management. This is particularly true for OSCAR, because its primary agents are nonspecialist Marines and it targets not only specific skills but also the culture of Marines in general. These results suggest that the overarching themes of OSCAR are concordant with the existing culture among Marines regarding combat stress management.

In closing this chapter, we emphasize a couple of specific findings from the focus groups that are particularly important because of their implications for the future design and implementation of combat and operational stress–control training programs. First, Marines frequently did not distinguish OSCAR from other combat stress–related programs, including more-general non–combat-related trainings on such topics as sexual harassment. In retrospect, it seems unreasonable to expect that they would, given the finding in the individual Marine survey that trainings related to combat stress were common, even among Marines in non–OSCAR battalions. It is highly likely that Marines draw on all of these trainings in forming their own attitudes and orientations to combat stress management. Therefore, consideration should be given to ensuring consistency across combat stress–control training programs provided to Marines, using a consistent set of concepts, terms, and expectations.

Second, where comments were made about specific aspects of OSCAR, the most commonly cited feature of the program was the color-coded stress continuum. Despite the fact that the stress continuum is not unique to OSCAR, some Marines clearly identified OSCAR with the continuum's color-coded gradations of stress. Moreover, even though participants were critical of the color-coding of stress, the continuum appeared to be well understood. It is likely that participants had the continuum in mind when they described how OSCAR provides a "common language" or "platform" for managing combat stress. These comments suggest that the barriers to more-effective combat stress management are not related to lack of education or knowledge among Marines but rather to a lack of tools, i.e., explicit terminology and official procedures, that Marines can use to address stress-related issues as they arise. Given the common appreciation of the serious nature of combat stress, a policy focus on providing tools, such as the continuum, might be an effective strategy for further improvements in combat stress management.

Limitations

In interpreting the results of the focus groups, it is important to consider the distinctive strengths and weaknesses of this method. A limitation is that the sample is not representative of the entire Marine Corps. This is particularly true in focus groups relative to other qualitative methods, such as one-on-one interviews, because the discussion in focus groups does not elicit the same information from each participant individually. The strength of these focus group discussions is that they provide windows into how people talk and reason about important "real-world" issues that affect their daily lives. Though particular opinions or attitudes expressed are not necessarily shared by all Marines, or even by all participants in a single focus group, the issues of concern that are mentioned are likely to be broadly shared. The qualitative data help elucidate the shared background that shapes the beliefs and actions of Marines with respect to combat stress response.

Summary

In concluding this chapter, we summarize the key themes identified from the focus groups as follows:

- Participants expressed some resistance to externally imposed combat stress programs.
- Participants perceived that the volume of combat stress–control training received is excessive, to the point that it might inadvertently sensitize Marines to stress.
- Participants did not always differentiate between OSCAR and other combat stress–management programs, instead mentally combining these programs into one broad category of programs related to psychological functioning.
- Combat stress was widely viewed as a very real concern.
- Participants emphasized the importance of peer relations and effective leadership in combat stress management.
- Participants preferred trainers with combat experience and "natural" mentors.
- Participants who had received OSCAR training reported valuing OSCAR as a "platform" for responding to combat stress problems that aligns well with military culture and routine.

CHAPTER SIX

Commanding Officers' Perceptions of OSCAR: Interviews with Battalion Commanding Officers

Battalion commanders have a uniquely valuable perspective on the management of combat-related stress in general and on OSCAR as a means of managing combat-related stress in particular. By the time Marines become commanders, they are likely to have combat leadership experience, to have observed a broad range of reactions to combat among Marines, and to have had responsibility for managing serious combat stress reactions. Their experience implementing OSCAR might provide valuable lessons. Moreover, battalion commanders are responsible for putting OSCAR into practice within their units. If the program does not meet their needs and fit their operational priorities, it is unlikely to be successfully implemented in the field.

For these reasons, the evaluation included a series of open-ended interviews with battalion commanders about their views of combat stress in general, their understanding of how OSCAR addresses their needs, and their recommendations for the future. One-on-one interviews were used rather than focus groups because of the difficulty scheduling a group of battalion commanders for a joint meeting and the desire on the part of the evaluators to be able to explore leaders' perspectives in greater detail than would be possible in a group setting.

This chapter describes the methods and results of one-on-one interviews with commanding officers of battalions that had received OSCAR training and discusses the implications of the findings.

Methods

Eighteen semistructured interviews were conducted by telephone with commanding officers of battalions that had received OSCAR training. The commanders were identified and recruited by the COSC office. All of the commanders had experience with OSCAR training, but 12 received training prior to their most recent deployment, while the remaining six received the training after their most recent deployment and thus did not have experience with OSCAR during a deployment. The questions that leaders were asked were similar to those posed to the focus groups discussed in the previous chapter. They covered commanders' views of combat stress, the best means of responding to combat stress, and their overall evaluation of OSCAR as a program.

Each interview was conducted by one of two RAND researchers over the telephone while another staff member took notes. Interviews were not audio recorded. Quotations provided below are based on the notes taken during the interview. The RAND evaluation team conducted thematic analyses of the interview notes.

Results

This section is organized according to the key themes and subthemes that emerged from the interviews. Key themes pertain to commanding officers' emphasis on the importance of effective leadership in stress-response management; perceptions that OSCAR reinforces principles of effective leadership; and views on the desired characteristics of OSCAR trainers, the Marines who should receive OSCAR training, and the ideal timing of OSCAR training. Illustrative quotes are provided for each theme and subtheme.

Commanders Emphasized the Importance of Effective Leadership in Combat and Operational Stress Management

The commander interviews were remarkable for their unanimity with respect to one dominant theme: that combat and operational stress management should be viewed primarily as a problem of effective leadership rather than medical intervention. According to this view, effective leaders create an environment of cohesion and high morale in the units they lead. Environments in cohesive units are seen as naturally conducive to positive responses to combat stress, including early identification of behavioral change, the absence of stigma related to care-seeking, and strong peer support that can obviate the need for removing affected people for medical care. Connections between effective leadership, unit cohesion, and combat stress management were highlighted by nearly all the commanding officers interviewed in such comments as the following:

> I never looked at it from a "How is OSCAR doing?" standpoint; saw it as a camaraderie and leadership issue. If a squad leader was good, it was almost automatic for the disclosure [of stress issues from young Marines] to come.

———

> I'm a big fan of positive command climate—a climate that's built on cohesion. Cohesion in and of itself is a force multiplier. I think cohesion perhaps is the best program, for lack of better terms, to help deal with [stress], before, during and after combat.

———

> Command climate, that sense you get when you step into a unit—and you just know it in your bones when you step in there. We tend to think of accountability as top-down, but the most important kind of accountability is peer-to-peer. It empowers people at both levels. Combat and operational stress is a unit disease, and each unit's experience is peculiar to that unit. Even in Iraq, the experiences were all [very different] depending on the unit. Dealing with those things is much better done peer-to-peer at the lower level. Healing [takes place best] at these levels.

———

It's good leadership—leaders or peers who are aware of operational stress in their peers and themselves—"seeing one of their brothers hurting and sitting down and talking about it"— not psychological professionals.

Commanders value effective stress management partly because they believe that, when a unit responds effectively to a Marine who is showing signs of stress, the response itself feeds back positively into improved cohesion and morale:

Again, a significant impact, because people believe that their unit cares about them, and that everyone gets treated fairly and equally. Whether it's PTS [posttraumatic stress] or financial issues. When people assist you when you have a challenge, it helps with unit cohesion.

————

[OSCAR] reinforces unit cohesion that already exists. People who have lived the same experiences as you foster cohesion, breed loyalty to one another.

Commanders View OSCAR as Consistent with Effective Leadership

This broad view of combat stress response informs the way that commanders view and understand the OSCAR program. Overwhelmingly, commanders voiced positive opinions of OSCAR because they view it as consistent with their existing principles of effective leadership:

I've found it's all tied to leadership traits. If you lack certain leadership traits, it tends to [manifest itself] in a positive climate or a negative climate. Whether it's the squad leader, or an old battalion commander [like me] who wasn't [an original] believer in the program. I became a believer in [OSCAR] after the training sessions. The program is in line with the leadership traits and principles . . . duty-bound to your subordinates . . . open communication, which sometimes the Marine Corps has a problem with. If you foster a command climate [at any level], people tend to lean on one another instead of hole up.

In discussing OSCAR, commanders cited four specific aspects of the program that they believe embody principles of effective leadership, which we briefly illustrate with quotations in this section.

OSCAR Normalizes Open Communication About Stressful Experiences and Psychological Reactions

[OSCAR] has a positive impact on improving communication. If a Marine opens up about something personal and is surprised by the support, like saying, "get out and go to your appointment" or "hey, don't have your meeting? Get out, it's important," [this] will increase confidence across the board about communication with leadership.

————

I think OSCAR forces you to talk about it. The number one thing leaders need to do is tell everybody—you're all going to get PTSD. It's not something that makes you special in any way. I think we all have to accept that we all have it. In my personal opinion, one of the responsibilities of a leader is to keep everyone in the fighting line. It's got to be a built-in component of leadership, of people understanding stress. There's nothing you can do about it. Mitigation, getting people back into the game, so to speak.

———

Biggest benefit is that has helped me create a cultural change . . . When I say "bring your problems forward," [junior Marines] think I'm full of crap. They might go 18 months and not ever believe me. Participants are forced to talk about themselves and their problems during the OSCAR training, and that changes the norm, shifts the paradigm.

OSCAR Provides a Common Language for Communicating About Stress

The other thing OSCAR does a fantastic job of is that it's a walking, talking human smoke detector for the unit. The connections it makes and provides, really at the NCO level, the language of a stress continuum. If you have team members who both come in and speak the same language, there's an immediate understanding, a common language. The fact that we're teaching the stress continuum is super important.

———

The OSCAR program gives you a foundation, a stress continuum model which I found to be effective. It's kind of cheesy, so you actually buy it. It's ingenious; to be brutally honest [the colors . . .] orange, yellow, red, etc. it provides a foundation for the Marine—he's either going to be resilient or not, and would the team make him resilient through those factors. Then with the mitigation part, it gives the squad a [way to treat] the Marine. The team shares the stress. I think the problem with the DoD in general [not so much OSCAR and the Marine Corps] is that everybody thinks that [OSCAR] is a medical program. But this is a leadership program.

———

We're using the terminology now—talk about if someone is "reacting," we are telling Marines that it's okay, we're not going to punish you. It has helped us frame the problem. We all know that, if you deploy twice, you are going to feel something, now we can distinguish more about what level of care they need: reacting versus very ill. Without that [framework], our response was slower, more drawn out. The previous command had a different perspective—I take it personally because I came back from Iraq with a lot of personal issues and no one understood what I was going through or what to do.

OSCAR Mobilizes and Reinforces Peer Support Without Involvement of External Resources or Authorities

In some cases, it almost feels like there is a glut. There are too many different external programs that it is hard for Marines to choose. OSCAR is internal and can be deployed down to the squad level. These young guys are more willing to discuss things with someone who knows their day-to-day lives.

———

Take home message was, "If there is a Marine sobbing in the portajohn, I want the guy in the next portajohn to knock and say, "hey, I can hear you. . . . What can we do?" To have the Marines understand that what is happening to the [sobbing] guy is a biological reaction —it is cortisol spike or something triggered in the amygdala, not weakness.

———

OSCAR provides a great forum at the unit level to discuss PTSD or stress as real and how to be on the lookout for it. OSCAR is a route for training Marines to recognize stress conditions on the lowest possible level, right along with other life-saving training. Likes to use the statistics that show that "a Marine treated in the unit is more likely to stay in the unit."

OSCAR Focuses on Readiness, Not Vulnerability to Stress

There is a singular goal to OSCAR—to keep a Marine in the fight. For those individuals who are unable to stay in the fight, to most rapidly return him to the fight. OSCAR's designed to keep your guys in the fight. It's not a charity organization; it's not something to feel bad for. Mission readiness.

———

The OSCAR program, as it is currently being implemented, has absolutely minimized the number of individuals we've had to evacuate out of theater. Most of it never leaves the unit level. He's able to have the support he needs within his battalion. We're talking dozens of individual Marines over the course of the year who didn't have to be removed from their unit to deal with stress. That's pretty significant in this counterinsurgency fight. Twelve individuals in a unit is a pretty big deal.

———

First and foremost is the combat readiness of the unit. That's my understanding of the purpose behind OSCAR. By having the Marines look out for each other and address issues early on, they can address issues in the combat theater.

—————

The reality is, it's just stress control. The signs and indicators and warning, that somebody has a problem, are no different whether the stress is coming from combat, or spousal abuse, child abuse, etc. All those additional stressors are going to come into play. How you come by the stress, frankly, is not relevant. OSCAR is about keeping the Marine in the fight, and out of the penalty box, so to speak. All of those things that can cause a Marine to be taken off line can be handled by stress control.

Commanders' Views of OSCAR Personnel and Training

Commanders were asked their opinions on the appropriate personnel for OSCAR (trainers and team members) and the content and timing of OSCAR training, and their answers were generally consistent with their broader views of the program. Given the emphasis on OSCAR skills as general leadership skills, the commanders advocated greater institutionalization of the program into standard operational training. Although there was a strong consensus regarding who should provide the training and the content of the training, there remained some disagreement about who should be trained.

Characteristics of OSCAR Trainers

Commanders were concerned that OSCAR trainers without combat experience would not command sufficient respect among Marines to convincingly advocate for the program. Commanders were particularly skeptical that Marines would relate positively to psychologists teaching them about combat stress and seeking mental health care because they had not themselves had to go through it. The ideal OSCAR trainer, according to several commanders, is someone who has extensive combat experience, might have actually been seriously wounded, and has gone on to have a successful career within the Marine Corps. Such a trainer would not only convey the information but show through example what is possible, which would make those lessons more likely to be effective:

The key to the whole thing is discussing active examples, and it must be someone with credibility. I recommend that, because unfortunately we have a growing population of Wounded Warriors, there might be some people there who could [be OSCAR leaders]. Not everyone would be qualified, but some would be perfect. I think there might be a population there that might want to stay on active duty, guys with missing legs, etc. Educate and train the heck out of them, but the credibility is automatically there—that would be powerful.

—————

The selection of the master trainer is key, and who rolls it out. The guy who's got to roll it out is the four-time-deployment sergeant who's gone out and [served] and whose career is continuing and ongoing because of the things that have troubled him. He's done it; he's wearing the combat action ribbon and has the street credibility to roll this thing out. The Marines [want to be like him]. The worst possible combination is a chaplain in uniform but not of that culture—it [won't stick]. The culture will probably reject the training from that person.

Recipients of OSCAR Training

Commanders were divided in their recommendations for who should receive training to fill the role of OSCAR team member. The divisions can be attributed to different ways that commanders balance three interrelated issues: the value of designating official OSCAR mentors or team members, the potential risk of oversensitization to stress, and the need for generalized knowledge and common expectations regarding stress and stress response across all ranks.

As discussed above, a key component of OSCAR is the selection of a group of NCOs to be trained to serve as team members, i.e., in a quasi-official role as a nonprofessional contact for Marines experiencing stress reactions. The role is quasi-official in the sense that the team members are identified and trained as individuals, but their activities are meant to be informal so that they can be approached without fear of stigma. The concern among some commanders is that it is unrealistic to expect Marines to turn to a designated team member or mentor for this type of support. For instance, consider the following:

> I believe that the individuals choose who their mentors are [you can't assign someone a mentor—it happens organically]. They're willing to go to them. And that's not always the case with the people we identify in the order. If I'm not religious—I'm not going to the chaplain. If I'm a PFC, I'm not going to the XO—there's no way. I see a flaw in the program in that we [need to] designate people to be the belly button at the very lower levels.

For some commanders, the idea that OSCAR principles are part of effective leadership leads to the suggestion that the training should be limited to commanders, rather than spread throughout the corps. These commanders remain concerned about the competence of non-professionals to make appropriate triage decisions:

> To empower the commander, to not become prescriptive as to how and specifically how we need to handle it. That's a road you don't want to go down on for future conflicts. Psychological injuries are very real, but there's also a great room for interpretation, whereas a physical injury is much easier to diagnose and treat. [It's easier to prescribe treatments for physical injuries than psychological injuries because there's less variability in how they manifest.] Keep the ball in the commander's court as much as possible.

The suggestion that OSCAR training should be limited to higher-level officers was a minority opinion. More commonly, commanders suggested the opposite strategy: training a much broader range of personnel, with the specific contents and format of the training tailored for different ranks and leadership roles. The reasons for these suggestions were in line with the opinions discussed above, i.e., that the impact of combat stress on readiness is best minimized by spreading knowledge of combat stress, setting expectations for recovery consistently, and providing a common language for talking about combat stress reactions.

The reason why I bring that up is that we absolutely need to push this type of training, preventive training, down to a more junior level than most people kind of think about it. The Marines, or the majority, still live in the barracks because they tend to be young single guys and gals. We tend to think we know what's going on in the barracks, the vaunted Marine Corps discipline and all that, but the reality is we don't. We really need young guys who have the maturity and wherewithal to accept this training and apply it quite effectively.

Timing of OSCAR Training

OSCAR training is typically provided to a battalion one time, immediately prior to deployment. Commanders, with a broader focus on stress response over the long term, suggested that the training could be more integrated with other types of training related to stress and psychological health, with multiple trainings tailored to specific stages of the deployment cycle:

> I think it's something you always want to work on, coming a month before we deployed was OK, but for a reserve unit you might think about doing the OSCAR training right after they're activated. They could have used some of those [stress] skills during the initial five-month training period [before deployment, after activation]. To have an introduction to OSCAR during the mobilization process might be good, then come back around the month before deployment and give them one extra dose. The stressors will be a little different, and you can focus first on the transition from civilian to military, away from their families, and then the second session would be on combat stressors, seeing people die.

Several commanders expressed concern about the fate of OSCAR after the end of the wars in Afghanistan and Iraq, when the need for combat stress management becomes less pressing. On the one hand, commanders would like to see the training institutionalized so that combat stress–response management would become a recognized and valued skill rather than an optional adjunct to combat training. Institutionalizing OSCAR during peacetime was viewed as a challenging problem:

> OSCAR is going to face challenges as we draw down from Afghanistan—could be seen as just a part of that, harder to sell.

———

> Yes, but I'd be worried about [as the war winds down, general reduction in resources, changing priorities] squeezing [OSCAR] out. But, [I think Marines] need to stay prepared for war, [including operational stress], even when not at war—just like combat training continues during peace time.

———

> OSCAR should be a program of record. Headquarters threw out a program that had a backbone but without all the details firmed up. Next it should become a program that is

"inspectable," that you can hold people accountable for, more institutionalized, or else it will die.

On the other hand, commanders were also concerned that OSCAR not become a "check-the-box program," meaning a program that people go through simply because it is required and without any appreciation for its intrinsic value:

> However, the challenge is going to be the implementation of the programs. Does it become a check in the box, or is it truly important? As we start normalizing in our operational tempo in the next ten years, I think there's always the potential for that to just become another requirement. Our advisers and senior leader advisers need to recognize that it's important.

Finally, several commanders also suggested a need for postdeployment training that would focus on the transition back into civilian life:

> We have to figure out the five days when you first get home, or some kind of stopping point between coming out of combat and coming home. Somewhere in the middle, there needs to be some time there where commanders have the ability to have some time with their Marines. It needs to come from the guys with the shared experience, to deal with issues that can be headed off before they head home. The five-day period when you come home [between leaving theater and coming home] needs to be used, always. The half-day rest, etc. And we need to provide this for the families as well. When the guys go on 30-day leave after their five days have passed, the command needs to stay intact so the guys know who they can relate to [and call on]. Don't rush guys off to school; don't [disband the command] too early after coming home from theater. That's the way to do it.

———

> The postdeployment piece needs to be better. Needs to be part of preparing for combat, and mitigating it [operational stress] during combat, but then it falls off, need to mitigate effects in the long term.

This suggestion is interesting because it reflects a desire by commanders to have a positive impact on stress response beyond the battlefield. Undoubtedly, these commanders are affected by reports of high levels of psychological distress among Marines and other service members that emerge after rather than during deployment. Application of the OSCAR principles to training for postdeployment stressors might be a valuable strategy.

Conclusions

The views of combat stress and OSCAR among battalion commanders are remarkably similar to those expressed by Marines in the focus groups. There is a common underlying conceptual model in which combat stress response is seen as an unavoidable and serious consequence of war and the response to people suffering from reactions to stress is seen as an important dimension of unit functioning. Both commanders and ordinary Marines emphasize that unit cohesion and morale set the stage for effective response to combat stress, which is better accomplished through peer-to-peer support than through specialized mental health intervention. Both commanders and Marines do not deny the reality of stress reactions but try to normalize them as expectable.

Not surprisingly, commanders tend to emphasize the leadership perspective, drawing direct connections between general leadership functions and internal dynamics of battalions. In doing so, they echo long-standing conceptions of the role of leadership in establishing group cohesion in order to improve effectiveness (Shils and Janowitz, 1948; Wessely, 2006). The research literature also supports the positive effect that unit cohesion can have on resilience to the psychological stressors of war (Bartone, 2006; Dickstein et al., 2010) and stigma related to mental health problems (Wright et al., 2009).

Finally, commanders expressed concern that it will be difficult to maintain OSCAR during peacetime. These commanders expect that the focus on combat stress reactions will decrease when Marines are not involved in actual combat. Most would like to see the lessons from Operations Enduring Freedom and Iraqi Freedom incorporated into normal practice within the Marine Corps, but they also fear that these lessons will be lost when the issues of combat stress lose their immediacy. Specific suggestions regarding how to accomplish this were varied and nonspecific. However, the institutionalization of combat stress–management training by providing it routinely and requiring mastery of the content as a core skill was widely endorsed.

Limitations

In interpreting findings from the interviews, it is important to consider the distinctive strengths and weaknesses of this method. Similar to the focus groups, a limitation is that the sample is not representative of battalion commanders across the entire Marine Corps. The strength of these interviews is that they provide detail-rich information on how commanding officers view the OSCAR program, which aspects of the program they value, and which aspects they consider in need of improvement.

Summary

In summary, key findings from the interviews with commanding officers include the following:

- Commanding officers acknowledged that combat stress is a real concern for Marines.
- Commanding officers emphasized the importance of effective leadership in combat stress management.
- Commanding officers perceived that OSCAR is consistent with principles of effective leadership in that it
  - normalizes open communication about stressful experiences and psychological reactions
  - provides a common language for communicating about stress
  - mobilizes and reinforces peer support without involvement of external resources or authorities
  - focuses on readiness, not vulnerability to stress.

- Commanders commonly espoused the following views regarding OSCAR personnel and training:
    - Ideally, an OSCAR trainer would have a history of extensive combat experience and might have actually been seriously wounded and gone on to have a successful career within the Marine Corps.
    - OSCAR training should be given to all Marine Corps leaders down to the level of squad leader, rather than limited to select NCOs and officers, and training should be tailored to Marines of different ranks.
    - OSCAR training should be conducted routinely to maintain skills, regardless of the deployment schedule (e.g., provide training on an annual basis).

CHAPTER SEVEN

Conclusions and Recommendations

OSCAR was designed to bridge the gap between specialty medical care for stress-related mental health problems and combat operations, where extremes of stressful experience are inevitable. This gap has been recognized for many years as a source of conflict, confusion, and inefficiency, rooted in fundamental differences in orientation between mental health professionals and military operational leaders. Two of the primary goals of mental health professionals are to identify and treat people with clinically significant psychiatric conditions. However, from the operational perspective, treatment involves isolation of someone from his or her unit and a focus on failure rather than peer support, which maintains unit morale, cohesion, and readiness. The OSCAR program represents the cutting edge of a long line of organizational innovations that aim to integrate these competing interests.

OSCAR integrates in two directions, bringing mental health professionals into field operations on a day-to-day basis and training nonmedical Marines in basic techniques of identifying potentially serious combat stress reactions. The integration of mental health professionals is accomplished by stationing care providers in forward positions where they share the environment of the people they treat. The training of nonmedical Marines is accomplished by selecting a team of key people for predeployment training to serve as informal resources for stress management outside the chain of command. The intent is that the team members will be more approachable than senior officers or medical personnel for average Marines who might have combat-related stress problems.

OSCAR was first introduced in the Marine Corps in 1999 and evolved over time as it gained traction with Marine Corps leaders. As of 2012, OSCAR was mandated across the Marine Corps. Our evaluation of OSCAR was conducted close to the end of this period, between 2010 and 2012, so that it is relevant to a relatively recent version of the program. In the remainder of this chapter, we review the key findings from the evaluation and offer actionable recommendations to improve OSCAR's ability to meet its primary objective of enhancing combat and operational stress control among Marines. In interpreting the findings and recommendations from this evaluation, bear in mind that, since this evaluation was designed and conducted, the OSCAR program might have undergone changes in its design and implementation that would not have been captured in our findings. Thus, our findings apply primarily to the impacts of the OSCAR program from March 2010 through October 2012.

Summary of the Evaluation Results

OSCAR Increases the Use of Support for Stress Problems, but There Was No Evidence of an Impact on Marines' Mental Health Status

The quantitative component of the evaluation suggests that OSCAR increased use of peers, leaders, and corpsmen as resources for stress-related problems but did not find evidence of an effect on the use of specialized mental health services. OSCAR's effects on support-seeking behavior persisted after adjustment for a wide array of baseline characteristics and deployment experiences, including exposure to combat, peritraumatic reactions, and deployment stressors, which increases confidence that these findings reflect an increase in willingness to seek support for stress problems as intended by the designers of OSCAR. However, given the possibility of residual confounding of OSCAR with battalion type, it is also possible that the differences in support-seeking observed between the OSCAR-trained and control battalions actually reflect differences in unmeasured need for help caused by the more-intensive combat experiences of Marines in the OSCAR-trained battalions, which were nearly all infantry, relative to the control battalions, which were all service support.

At the same time, this evaluation did not find evidence that OSCAR had an impact on mental health stigma or mental health outcomes. Marines in the battalions in which OSCAR was implemented were no less likely than those in control battalions to report mental health problems, such as PTSD, depression, or substance use, on the T2 survey. Firm conclusions regarding OSCAR's effectiveness are difficult to draw given that the lack of significant effects on several key outcomes has multiple possible causes. These causes include the study's methodological limitations—namely, the limited precision to detect significant effects that resulted from statistical adjustments for confounds and the clustering of observations within battalions; the comparison of OSCAR to a "stress-control-training-as-usual" control condition, which might have left less room for OSCAR to exert an incremental benefit on stress-related attitudes and mental health outcomes; possible variability in implementation of OSCAR across battalions, which was suggested by variation in outcomes across OSCAR-trained battalions and anecdotal reports from our points of contact (POCs) in the Marine Corps; and the possibility that OSCAR, even if implemented consistently and with fidelity to the program's design, does not improve stress-related attitudes, help-seeking behavior, and mental health outcomes relative to the other types of stress-control training Marines received in the non–OSCAR-trained (control) battalions. This last possibility should be considered in light of the fact that none of the components of OSCAR has an evidence base and in the context of the broader landscape of prevention programs, which is remarkable for the lack of effective prevention programs (IOM, 2014; Meredith et al., 2011).

Also of interest was the finding that OSCAR team members, who are Marine Corps leaders without professional mental health training who have been trained to serve as designated POCs for Marines experiencing stress reactions, did not report an increase in consultations from Marines after OSCAR training. This might indicate a potential limitation of the OSCAR model. If Marines do not make use of the OSCAR team members, then the team members might not contribute to the program. One possible reason for this finding was illuminated in some of the qualitative data, in which Marines indicated that having designated mentors would not be effective because Marines would not seek out help from someone whom they did not already know and trust.

Marines View Combat and Operational Stress as a Serious but Surmountable Problem

In contrast with anecdotal accounts from prior historical periods, findings from the qualitative components of this evaluation suggested that Marines were informed about potential mental health consequences of combat and operational stress, recognized it as a serious problem, and shared a basic conceptual model for how it should be managed. Moreover, this shared model reflects many of the same principles that underlie the design of OSCAR. Stressors of war are seen as inevitable and universally troubling but unlikely to cause lasting psychological illness in the large majority of people. In many cases, informal and mutual social support among Marines was perceived as helpful in mitigating the impact of stressors, obviating the need for medical intervention. Identification of Marines whose reactions cross a threshold of clinical significance, where medical intervention is indicated, is understood to be an important though difficult task, and recovery from psychological injuries is expected. The qualitative findings converged with findings from the surveys, in which Marines endorsed positive expectations for recovery from the long-term effects of combat stressors. It is likely that this shared model derives from trainings that Marines have received on combat and operational stress control and is not distinctive of OSCAR.

At the same time, Marines also recognized the difficulties of seeking help for combat-related stress. Concerns that stigma associated with psychological problems prevents Marines from seeking mental health services were frequently voiced in the focus groups and the commander interviews. Some participants argued that stigma could never be eliminated, while some were hopeful that new generations of Marines are more accustomed to mental health care and thus less likely to stigmatize those who seek it. Stigma was considered to be a serious reputational threat with negative career consequences within the Marine Corps. Concern with stigma among Marines contributes to the perceived importance of informal sources of support, such as trusted peers, as opposed to medical services. In the surveys, endorsement of the use of informal sources of support was common.

OSCAR Is Perceived as a Useful Tool for Combat and Operational Stress Control

Although we did not detect significant effects of OSCAR on most of the outcomes examined in the quantitative surveys, the overall perceptions of OSCAR expressed by battalion commanders in the qualitative interviews were generally positive. Given the alignment between the principles behind the design of OSCAR and the cultural models of combat and operational stress among Marines, this is not surprising. In particular, battalion commanders valued OSCAR because the program fit into their broader understanding of their roles as leaders. Emphasizing this point, one of the key informants said that he was initially skeptical of OSCAR because he was wary of overemphasizing mental health problems and individualized psychiatric treatment for PTSD. After the OSCAR training, however, he came to value the program as a framework for managing combat and operational stress on a unit-wide basis employing principles of group leadership, such as cohesion, morale, and mutual support among peers.

Participants in the focus groups were somewhat ambivalent about combat stress–response training in general, and many complained that they had received too many training courses on the topic. However, they also voiced support for the principles that underlie OSCAR—in particular, the emphasis on peer support and avoidance of medical intervention through early identification and management of stress and mental health problems.

Potential Problems Were Identified

Other potential problems with OSCAR were also identified. First, although the term *OSCAR* was widely recognized by our respondents, it was not clear that they distinguished clearly between OSCAR and other training programs related to combat and operational stress control. In fact, some respondents seemed to lump OSCAR together with a broad range of training programs that included, for instance, training related to sexual harassment. Many complained about having received too much training on combat and operational stress control. These complaints might not reflect problems with the OSCAR program but with its integration into the overall combat stress–response training program in the Marine Corps.

Second, respondents made frequent recommendations related to the timing of OSCAR training. Some suggested that additional training was needed and that it should be organized around the deployment cycle. Others expressed the concern that, if OSCAR is tied only to the deployment cycle, it will not be maintained during peacetime. Annual trainings, regardless of deployment, were recommended as a way to keep Marines in a state of readiness for future combat deployments.

Finally, in the individual Marine survey, we also found evidence of significant variation in outcomes across OSCAR-trained battalions, potentially indicating that the implementation of OSCAR was not consistent across the battalions that received it. Anecdotal evidence from our POCs within the Marine Corps further reinforced the notion that OSCAR was implemented inconsistently across battalions.

Recommendations

Collectively, findings from the four components of this evaluation indicate that, although OSCAR has had success in obtaining the support of Marine Corps leadership, it has not fulfilled its mission of improving many of the key outcomes that it was designed to affect. Thus, this evaluation did not find evidence of OSCAR's effectiveness that would support the continuation of OSCAR in its current form. In recommending a way forward for the Marine Corps in its efforts to manage combat and operational stress, we rely on findings from this evaluation's qualitative components, other research, and best practices for program improvement and implementation.

Informed by this evaluation's findings of reports of excessive stress-response training, we recommend that the Marine Corps review all of its combat and operational stress–control training programs, including OSCAR, with the goal of streamlining these programs to reduce duplication of effort. In revising the approach to combat and operational stress–response training, we suggest identifying potential solutions that might increase the effectiveness of such training (e.g., modifying implementation approaches or modifying target population), taking into account program participants' perspectives on features of OSCAR that were noted to be positive and suggestions for improvement. Next, consistent with best practices for program improvement and implementation (Ryan et al., 2014), we recommend small-scale pilot-testing of selected solutions to determine feasibility and effectiveness in targeting the intended outcomes. Then, if the small-scale pilot test proves promising, the solutions could gradually be scaled up. If the tested solutions do not show evidence of feasibility and effectiveness on a small scale, the Marine Corps might wish to discontinue its investments in OSCAR and instead invest resources in other psychological health policies and programs that already have a stronger evidence base with respect to their impact on psychological health. These recommendations are described in greater detail below.

Because none of these recommendations has been formally tested, we do not know the extent to which their adoption will positively affect combat and operational stress management in the Marine Corps. Moreover, some of the recommendations might be very difficult to implement in light of organizational, policy, regulatory, and budgetary constraints. Thus, the recommendations offered here should be viewed as suggestive rather than prescriptive. Ultimately, the Marine Corps and other stakeholders (e.g., the Defense Centers of Excellence for Psychological Health and Traumatic Brain Injury [DCoE]) will need to determine which recommendations are feasible to implement and likely to produce their intended benefits.

Recommendation 1. Review and Streamline Marine Corps Combat and Operational Stress–Control Training Programs

The evaluation results highlighted the excess of combat and operational stress–control training received by Marines, suggesting the need for a more streamlined approach to this type of training. The evaluation also shed light on Marine Corps leaders' perceptions of positive features of OSCAR and features of OSCAR that might have undermined its potential to mitigate combat stress. In integrating and streamlining combat and operational stress–control training programs, the Marine Corps might wish to consider retaining or strengthening the positive features of OSCAR and redesigning or eliminating features that were less positively perceived.

Recommendation 1.1. Identify and Reduce Duplication of Effort in Combat and Operational Stress–Control Trainings

The major complaint voiced by Marines in the focus groups was that they had received too much training related to combat stress. In most cases, Marines did not distinguish between OSCAR training as a specific program and other combat and operational stress-related trainings that they had received. This anecdotal evidence was backed up by the surveys, which showed that even members of battalions that had not received the OSCAR training had, on average, about two prior training sessions related to combat and operational stress. Not only is it likely that there is duplication of effort in these multiple trainings; it is also possible that Marines are being given different messages about stress response through their official trainings. These findings dovetail with those of a recent scan of all traumatic brain injury and psychological health programs sponsored or funded by DoD in which the decentralized nature of information about programs, which contributes to a lack of information-sharing and redundancy of efforts across programs, was identified as a barrier to maximizing program effectiveness (Weinick et al., 2011). We recommend a thorough review of the concepts and methods of combat stress–response training programs that would align the content and rationalize the scheduling of training in this area across the Marine Corps. This recommendation coincides with a similar call from the USMC Behavioral Health Branch to have better integration across USMC Behavioral Health programs.

Recommendation 1.2. Enhance the Use of a Common Language for Concepts Related to Combat and Operational Stress Control Across Combat and Operational Stress Control Programs

We also recommend that, in the process of reviewing and streamlining combat and operational stress–control training, planners pay attention to consistency in the concepts and specific language across training programs and the procedures that are taught. This recommendation reflects the goal mentioned above of reducing duplication of effort, and it also reflects the findings from the qualitative analysis that OSCAR was valued because of its being a shared language for talking about and managing combat stress response. Thus, this language would ideally be widely, if not universally, shared among Marines. A common language coupled with a common set of procedures taught through a consistent set of training courses is important for maximizing the effectiveness of combat and operational stress–control training.

Recommendation 1.3. Ensure That Combat and Operational Stress–Control Program Trainers Have Combat Experience

We recommend that particular attention be paid to maintaining a group of qualified combat and operational stress–control program trainers who have combat experience and are effective at communicating the value of the training to their fellow Marines. This recommendation echoes the current OSCAR training guidelines, which specify a preference for trainers with combat experience. The credibility of a source is a powerful determinant of the persuasiveness of the message communicated by the source, and research has consistently shown that expertise and trustworthiness are the two key dimensions of credibility (Pornpitakpan, 2004). Findings from the qualitative components of the evaluation indicate that, in the eyes of Marines, combat experience and prior experience dealing with serious combat stress or injury are critical indicators of expertise and trustworthiness insofar as combat and operational stress management is concerned. Research participants repeatedly emphasized the importance of using trainers with personal experience in combat stress. Focus group participants and battalion commanders both spoke about the ideal OSCAR trainer as a Marine who had been in combat and had prior experience dealing with serious combat stress or injury. These comments indicate the value that Marines put on the personal and experience-based authority of their fellow Marines over and above that of professionals who might have learned about combat stress in classes or through clinical practice but who have not experienced combat firsthand.

Recommendation 2. Identify Potential Changes to the Design and Implementation of Combat and Operational Stress–Control Training

Ideas about potential changes to the design and implementation of combat and operational stress–control training that might increase the effectiveness of such training can come from many sources, including program participants, implementation literature, and other programs. In this section, we suggest potential changes to this training based on the findings from this evaluation.

Recommendation 2.1. Consider Providing Combat and Operational Stress–Control Training to All Marines in the Chain of Command, Down to the Level of Squad Leader

By design, OSCAR team members are intended to be POCs outside the chain of command for consultation related to psychological stress, with the idea that they would not be required by their official roles to respond in a particular way, such as ordering someone to seek medical attention. As such, battalion commanders are instructed to select OSCAR team members based on qualities that make them effective "natural mentors," i.e., people who are respected for their integrity and trustworthiness who would be effective in giving advice because of their personal characteristics, not their rank. However, these potential advantages have to be balanced against the suggestion by participants in the focus groups and the interviews that Marines are unlikely to seek out advice of someone they do not know just because he or she has been designated as an OSCAR team member. In fact, the designation of a person as an OSCAR team member might make him or her less approachable because he or she has an official status, even if that official status is meant to be informal.

Our recommendation is that, in streamlining the existing suite of combat and operational stress–control training programs, consideration be given to providing the streamlined training program to leaders within the chain of command down to the level of squad leader, rather than informal mentors. According to the findings from the qualitative component of the evaluation, the informal status of a team member does not seem compatible with the Marine Corps culture of clearly designated chains of command and reporting responsibilities. Marines can make use of informal supports by consulting with their peers but might be as resistant to consulting a designated OSCAR team member as they would to consulting a medical professional or other superior officer. Designating a respected individual as an OSCAR team member might have the unintended consequence of making him or her less approachable for average Marines. In addition, there was no evidence in the quantitative component of the evaluation that Marines sought out OSCAR team members more than they did prior to the OSCAR program. This finding is further evidence that the designation of a person as an OSCAR team member did not have the intended effect of providing an additional gateway to support or treatment for combat-related stress problems.

As an alternative to designating a small group of people as representatives of the program, we recommend providing training across a much broader group of small-group leaders so that individual consultations are not stigmatized and the effectiveness of response to combat-related stress will not be compromised. If many or all small-group leaders are qualified to respond to combat stress problems among Marines and understand that responding effectively is part of their leadership competence, then asking for help or advice would not identify a person as help-seeking and could therefore avoid or reduce the fear of being stigmatized. Training all leaders would be consistent with the approach taken by the Marine Corps' suicide prevention program, "Never Leave a Marine Behind," in which all NCOs and officers in the Marine Corps are required to complete annual training on suicide prevention (U.S. Marine Corps, 2012).

Recommendation 2.2. Integrate Combat and Operational Stress–Control Training into the Deployment Cycle and Maintain It Regularly Among Nondeploying Troops

Regularizing combat and operational stress–control training, with annual trainings and booster sessions, can help to make responses to combat and operational stress a normal and routine part of Marine Corps life rather than an exceptional event. Booster training sessions are recommended in guidelines for enhancing the fidelity of program implementation in that they help to prevent deterioration of skills learned in training and drift from the program protocol, i.e., inclusion of training components that are not part of the program protocol or inadvertent exclusion of components that are part of the program protocol (Bellg et al., 2004; Saks and Belcourt, 2006). This was also a common recommendation from the battalion commanders who see routinization of effective stress response as an important component of their leadership skill. Maintaining readiness with respect to combat stress response during peacetime was flagged by several battalion commanders as a priority at risk of being overlooked in the drawdown from the wars in Afghanistan and Iraq.

Recommendation 3. Pilot Test Changes to Combat and Operational Stress–Control Training

Consistent with best practices for program development and implementation (Ryan et al., 2014), changes to the combat and operational stress–control training program should be pilot-tested on a small scale to determine their feasibility and effectiveness with respect to their impact on key outcomes. If results of the pilot test are promising, the program's implementation can be gradually expanded and assessed to identify and correct challenges of implementation that inevitably accompany program expansion. Borrowing from the best practices and recommendations from the National Institutes of Health Behavior Change Consortium (Bellg et al., 2004), we recommend examination of the following components of the program's implementation: (1) *delivery*, or the extent to which the program is delivered as intended according to the protocol (i.e., does the program as delivered cover all of the aspects of the protocol and convey them accurately to trainees?), (2) *receipt*, or the program participants' understanding of the content covered and ability to apply it in real-world situations, and (3) *enactment*, or the participants' application of the content to real-world scenarios that arise during deployment or in other military contexts with high levels of operational stress (i.e., do program participants successfully apply the program's principles and practices when needed and refrain from applying practices that are not part of the program?).

If the pilot test is not successful, then the Marine Corps might wish to revise the program based on process improvement data collected during the pilot test and test the revised version. Alternatively, the Marine Corps might prefer to abandon this approach to stress-control training and consider shifting its investments in psychological health to other policies and programs that have a stronger evidence base. For example, more resources could be invested in the implementation and dissemination of evidence-based treatments for PTSD and MDD in the Military Health System.

Recommendation 4. Expand the Evidence Base Regarding Operational Stress Management

A great deal of work remains to be done in order to learn the lessons from the initial implementation of OSCAR and use those lessons to improve combat and operational stress management in the Marine Corps. In particular, as the drawdown from Afghanistan continues, there is an opportunity to focus attention on further improving the design of combat and operational stress–control training programs.

Recommendation 4.1. Examine Patterns of Support-Seeking and Help-Seeking in More Detail

The findings from this study regarding support and help-seeking are puzzling in that we found an increase in seeking of support from informal sources in the OSCAR-trained battalions, but we also found that OSCAR team members did not report having had more consultations at postdeployment than prior to deployment. These findings suggest that the change in support-seeking might have occurred in unanticipated and unintended ways using pathways of support that are not formally part of OSCAR. Moreover, the nature of the support-seeking reported by Marines is not clear, and the decision process for selecting sources of support has not been examined. Information on the process for seeking support from informal sources and help from formal sources is critical to the continuing improvement of combat and operational stress–control systems.

Conclusion

Managing psychological reactions to stress in the context of military combat is an extremely challenging problem and has been the goal of continual policy innovation across the U.S. military for several generations. The OSCAR program represents an attempt to achieve this innovation in the Marine Corps, advancing principles of responding to combat stress rapidly with judicious use of medical treatment. Although we found no significant effects of OSCAR on stress-related attitudes and mental health outcomes, we found an increase in the use of resources, such as peers, leaders, and corpsmen, for stress-related problems, among Marines in OSCAR-trained battalions relative to those in control battalions. Collectively, the components of this evaluation indicate that OSCAR has not fulfilled its mission of improving combat and operational stress control but has nonetheless gained traction within the Marine Corps because of its high compatibility with Marine Corps culture. The evaluation results do not support continuation of OSCAR in its current form; however, they do yield lessons learned about positive features of OSCAR and opportunities for improvement in combat and operational stress–control training. We draw from suggestions from focus group participants and commanding officers, empirical findings from other research, and best practices for program implementation to recommend integrating and streamlining the Marine Corps' existing suite of combat and operational stress–control training programs and incorporating lessons learned from this evaluation in the development of the streamlined program. There are no quick fixes to addressing combat and operational stress and mental health problems, and much work remains to be done to address these problems.

Theoretical Background of OSCAR

Combat and Operational Stress Continuum

The Combat and Operational Stress Continuum model, hereafter referred to as the stress-continuum model, is the product of a working group convened in September 2007 that spanned the three MEFs (Chief of Naval Operations and Commandant of the Marine Corps, 2010). Working group participants included line commanders, senior enlisted leaders, chaplains, medical and mental health professionals, and HQMC policymakers. This model, which became the bedrock of all doctrine in psychological health and in combat and operational stress control in both the Marine Corps and Navy, describes responses to combat and operational stress along a spectrum of possible outcomes that range in severity from "adaptive coping" and "full readiness" to clinical mental disorders. The stress-continuum model (see Figure A.1) applies four possible categories to its continuum, color-coded as green ("ready"), yellow ("reacting"), orange ("injured"), and red ("ill").

An important departure of the stress-continuum model from previous conceptualizations of combat stress reactions is the addition of the concept of "stress injuries," a modification designed to bridge the gap between mild stress reactions at one end of the spectrum and clinical mental disorders at the other end (Nash, 2011). This modification, borrowed from the

Figure A.1
Marine Corps Combat and Operational Stress Continuum

Ready	Reacting	Injured	Ill

• Good to go
• Well trained
• Prepared
• Fit and tough
• Cohesive units, ready families
	• Distress or impairment
	• Mild, transient
	• Anxious or irritable
	• Behavior change
		• More-severe or persistent distress or impairment
		• Leaves lasting evidence (personality change)
			• Stress injuries that do not heal without intervention
			• Diagnosable
			  – PTSD
			  – Depression
			  – Anxiety
			  – Addictive disorder

Unit leader responsibility	Individual responsibility		Chaplain and medical responsibility

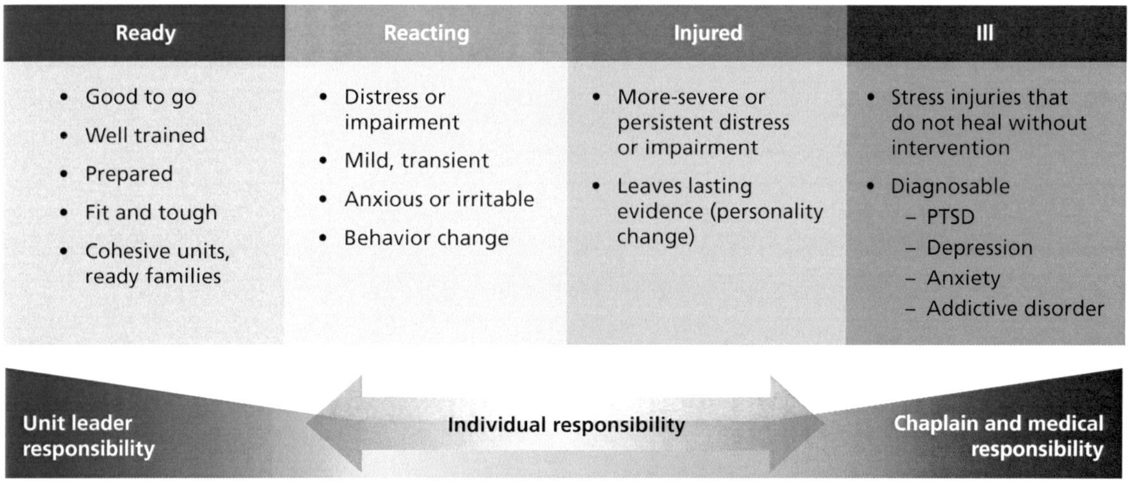

SOURCE: Chief of Naval Operations and Commandant of the Marine Corps, 2010.
RAND RR562-A.1

concept of physical injuries, reflects the recent transition of the Marine Corps and Navy to a more medicalized model of combat stress problems. The placement of stress reactions along a continuum was intended to emphasize the importance of identifying stress problems early in their development to prevent their escalation to more-severe stress reactions, e.g., to keep people who are merely "reacting" from progressing to the "injured" or "ill" zones. OSCAR team members are expected to be able to identify the stress-continuum zones of individual Marines in their units and be prepared to provide appropriate assistance, including referring them to the appropriate resources. For example, an OSCAR team member who identifies one of his or her Marines as being in the orange zone should strongly consider referring him or her to a chaplain or medical personnel.

Core Leader Functions

Building on the stress-continuum model, the Navy and Marine Corps identified five "core leader functions" to promote psychological health and build resilience (see Figure A.2) (Chief of Naval Operations and Commandant of the Marine Corps, 2010). All Navy and Marine Corps leaders, including but not limited to the officers and senior NCOs who receive training to become OSCAR team members, should (1) *strengthen* their Marines and sailors by fostering unit cohesion and exposing them to realistic training, (2) *mitigate* stress by ensuring adequate rest and removing unnecessary stressors, (3) *identify* signs of stress in their Marines and sailors, (4) *treat* stress with rest and restoration or referral to a chaplain or mental health provider, and (5) *reintegrate* Marines and sailors who have recovered from stress problems back into the unit. The first two of these functions, strengthen and mitigate, have long been emphasized in military doctrine on combat and operational stress control (Nash, Westphal, et al., 2010). The last

Figure A.2
Marine Corps Core Leader Functions

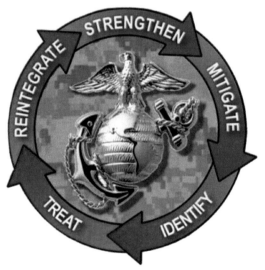

SOURCE: Naval Center for Combat and Operational
Stress Control, undated.
RAND RR562-A.2

three functions, identify, treat, and reintegrate, are more-recent additions to military doctrine on combat and operational stress control. These actions are further specified here:

- *Strengthen:* Leaders should help expand Marines' capacity for stress, making it more likely that they can withstand greater amounts of stress and still remain in the green and yellow zones.
- *Mitigate:* Leaders should pay attention to different sources of stress among their Marines, including not only combat-related problems but other concerns, such as finances, relationship problems, or health problems. The goal for leaders is to enable early recognition of possible problems and help Marines keep their overall stress levels manageable. This can be done by mitigating more-controllable stressors (e.g., conflicts with superiors) to conserve coping resources for less controllable stressors (e.g., seeing a fellow Marine injured in combat). Leaders can also mitigate stress problems by reducing stigma within the unit and demonstrating the possibility of learning from stressful experiences through posttraumatic growth. Leaders can do this by talking openly to the Marines in their units about stress problems, e.g., sharing their own experiences with stress, including healthy stress-management approaches and positive outcomes of these experiences; conveying an attitude of acceptance and encouragement to Marines in their units who are receiving help for stress problems; and generally modeling healthy attitudes and behaviors toward stress management.
- *Identify:* Leaders are expected to "know their Marines, i.e., be familiar with the typical mood, behavior, appearance, and body language of each of their Marines, so that they will be able to detect changes that might indicate a burgeoning stress problem. Following a mission, leaders are encouraged to use the after-action review, in which the unit members review the strengths and weaknesses of their performance, as an opportunity to look for behavioral changes in their Marines.
- *Treat:* If a leader notices signs of stress problems indicating that a Marine is in the yellow, orange, or red zone of the stress continuum, he or she is advised to take action, with the stipulation that "treating" is not meant to imply that unit leaders act as clinicians, but rather intervene early with a Marine exhibiting stress problems and help ensure that that Marine gets into clinical care. Leaders can intervene by
  - ensuring that physical needs are met, e.g., providing a period of rest
  - providing psychological first aid (Nash and Watson, 2012), which includes engaging with the Marine, providing safety and comfort, gathering information and providing practical assistance, and connecting the Marine with social supports and information on coping
  - referring anyone with an urgent need for medical attention to a mental health professional and facilitating mental health treatment adherence.
- *Reintegrate:* Leaders should mentor Marines who have experienced stress problems (and received mental health treatment) to prepare them to return to duty. An important element in reintegration is reducing the stigma related to seeking treatment.

Combat and Operational Stress First Aid

A set of psychological first aid techniques, COSFA, has been adapted for use in a military setting (Nash, Westphal, et al., 2010). The COSFA algorithm is the product of a collaborative effort among the Navy, Marine Corps, DCoE, and the Veterans Affairs National Center for PTSD (Nash, Westphal, et al., 2010). COSFA principles were designed to align with the guidelines for psychological first aid developed by the National Child Traumatic Stress Network and the National Center for PTSD (Brymer et al., 2006). The primary difference between COSFA and psychological first aid is that, in COSFA, the stress-continuum model informs decisions regarding when an intervention is needed, the type of intervention to provide, and assessment of recovery (Nash, Krantz, et al., 2011).

The procedures for COSFA closely resemble those used for physical first aid (Nash, 2006), again reinforcing the transition from a demedicalized model of combat and operational stress control to a more medicalized model. Although it is aimed primarily at facilitating recovery from orange-zone stress injuries, COSFA is part of the armamentarium of tools available for treating subclinical stress reactions and injuries in the yellow and orange zones of the stress continuum and preventing those outcomes from escalating to clinical disorders in the red zone. COSFA might be used in an emergency situation to keep someone safe until other interventions can be applied or, for less severe stress injuries, might be sufficient to restore someone to the green zone.

COSFA is intended to be a tool that leaders can use to perform the core leader functions of identify, treat, and reintegrate (Nash, Westphal, et al., 2010). Although leaders are expected to understand and implement COSFA when needed, the people deemed best suited to serve as its "champions, i.e., local experts in its implementation, are caregivers from various specialties, including chaplains, medical officers, corpsmen, RPs, and mental health professionals (Nash, Westphal, et al., 2010). This role assignment is consistent with the broader COSC-related prescription that medical and religious ministry personnel, who also serve as OSCAR extenders, should be a key resource in the treatment of orange-zone stress injuries.

COSFA consists of seven procedures or core components (Nash, 2011; Nash, Westphal, et al., 2010), delineated here:

1. *Check:* Check routinely for alterations in behavior that might indicate a combat stress problem. Ascertain whether there is a need for intervention, and continue to monitor and assess for stress problems that develop later or do not improve as expected.
2. *Coordinate:* Apprise leaders and family members of people who have sustained stress injuries of their status, request help and support from leaders and family members as needed, and follow up to make sure that appropriate help and support are provided.
3. *Cover:* Take action to protect someone suffering from acute distress or unusual changes in behavior, as well as other proximally situated people, until the distressed person resumes his or her typical level of functioning.
4. *Calm:* Help the distressed person lower his or her level of physiological arousal by performing deep breathing exercises and other relaxation techniques.
5. *Connect:* Following the occurrence of a stress reaction, injury, or illness, facilitate the provision of support from peers, family members, and other sources of social support to the person who suffered the reaction, injury, or illness. Offer support by listening and conveying reassurance.

6. *Competence:* Help the injured person perform competently in all areas and mentor him or her to achieve his or her full reintegration into the unit.

7. *Confidence:* Promote recovery of self-esteem; help the person regain the trust of his or her peers, others in the unit, and family members; and instill hope.

Pre- and Postassessment of January 2010 Operational Stress Control and Readiness Training[1]

Introduction

The OSCAR program is designed to embed mental health personnel within Marine Corps units and to increase the capability of Marines in officer and senior NCO roles to extend the reach of these mental health personnel by providing early recognition and intervention for Marines exhibiting signs of stress. As such, the Marines who take on this role as OSCAR "extenders" require specific training in operational stress control in order to achieve the central goals of the OSCAR program: to reduce stigma associated with stress responses and to facilitate early identification of stress reactions, injuries, and illnesses.

The first OSCAR training for extenders using newly redesigned materials occurred on January 21, 2010, at the Marine Corps base in Twenty-Nine Palms, California, and was presented by Battelle and sponsored by the Marine Corps Combat and Operational Stress Control (COSC) program. The training session lasted for six hours and addressed the importance of identifying and responding to stress problems, significant stressors that can lead to problems, and instruction in the proper response to stress problems. The training consisted of Power-Point-assisted presentations and role playing exercises. For half of the training, junior (E8 and below) and senior (E9 and above) leaders were separated into two training groups in different locations.

RAND researchers conducted an evaluation of this training to assess the general effectiveness of the newly developed curriculum materials being used for the first time.

Methods

To assess the training, we constructed pre and post surveys to be implemented among training participants. The survey content was developed based on review of the training materials and in cooperation with the Marine Corps COSC program, particularly Thomas Nash and William Gaskin. Topics covered in the pre- and posttraining surveys included:

- vignettes describing Marine behavior, with open-ended questions inquiring about next steps after concerning behavior is observed
- knowledge and preparedness to execute OSCAR responsibilities
- confidence in OSCAR-related skills

---

[1] Weinick et al. (2011). This report was prepared for the DCoE in 2010.

- perceptions regarding likely changes in the unit as a result of OSCAR training
- experiences during the training session.

We administered a 16-item pretraining survey and a 41-item posttraining survey (including a readministration of one ten-item battery from the pretraining survey) to identify how well prepared the trainees felt to meet their OSCAR obligations. The survey was administered in a completely deidentified, anonymous manner, with both surveys included in a single packet that the Marines retained during the training session. They placed their completed surveys in sealed envelopes and returned them to the RAND employee present at the training. No personal identifiers were requested. This project was approved by the RAND Human Subjects Protection Committee (HSPC).

We received 44 surveys from trainees, although no more than 43 trainees answered most individual questions.

The survey was designed and printed prior to last-minute changes made to the content of the training materials. As a result, a few of the questions that were included were no longer relevant to the training contents and are not included in this report. The full survey instrument is reproduced at the end of this appendix. Our posttraining survey was administered in conjunction with two other surveys of which the RAND team was not aware prior to the training date, one administered by Battelle and the other by the Marine Corps COSC program.

Results

Background Information

Approximately half of the respondents (56 percent) had participated in previous trainings to help them recognize the zones of the stress continuum and intervene to restore their own or their fellow Marines' mental and spiritual well-being. Of those responding, 70 percent were enlisted personnel; the remaining 30 percent were officers (data not shown).

Respondents' Sense of Preparedness

Prior to the training, approximately three-quarters of the respondents reported feeling less than "well prepared" for their OSCAR duties, including helping to restore the self-confidence of Marines recovering from stress injuries and teaching Marines in their units how to monitor and reduce each other's stress levels (see Table B.1). After the training, nearly all Marines reported feeling either "somewhat more prepared" or "much more prepared" in each of these areas. However, there were two areas of inquiry in which respondents were less likely to report that they were either somewhat or much more prepared after the training: helping Marines reintegrate into their units after being treated elsewhere for stress and knowing all of the resources available to help Marines in need of assistance. These areas might present potential opportunities for expansions or improvements in the training materials.

Table B.1
Preparedness to Carry Out OSCAR Expectations

	How Prepared Do You Feel							
	Before Training				After Training			
How Prepared Do You Feel to . . .	Very Unprepared, Somewhat Unprepared, or Somewhat Prepared		Well Prepared or Very Well Prepared		Less Prepared or About the Same		Somewhat More Prepared or Much More Prepared	
	n	%	n	%	n	%	n	%
Know how to recognize stress zones that require help?	32	74.4	11	25.6	2	4.7	41	95.4
Provide direct help to Marines who are in stress zones that place them at increased risk?	29	67.4	14	32.6	4	9.3	39	90.7
Identify Marines in stress zones that place them at risk for either failing to perform their duties or developing long-term stress illnesses?	31	72.1	12	27.9	1	2.3	42	97.7
Help restore the self-confidence of Marines who are recovering from stress injuries that briefly interfered with their job performance?	32	74.4	11	25.6	6	14.0	37	86.1
Teach Marines in your unit how to monitor each other's stress zones and help each other reduce stress?	31	72.1	12	27.9	5	11.6	38	88.4
Know which stress zones can be managed in the unit and which require referral to a mental health professional?	31	72.1	12	27.9	4	9.3	39	90.7
Help a Marine reintegrate into your unit after being treated somewhere else for stress?	34	79.1	9	20.9	12	28.6	30	71.4
Know all the resources available to help Marines in a high-stress zone, both in theater and at your home base?	34	79.1	9	20.9	10	23.3	33	76.7
Advise and support your unit leadership to prevent, recognize, and take care of stress injuries?	32	74.4	11	25.6	4	9.3	39	90.7

Knowledge of OSCAR Functions

Posttraining, all or nearly all respondents reported agreeing or strongly agreeing with the following statements (data not shown):

- "I understand my role as an OSCAR team member."
- "I am confident that I can identify someone with an orange-zone stress injury."
- "I am confident that I know what to do when a Marine is in the orange zone."

We also asked trainees to identify the core functions that all leaders should be able to perform in order to support Marine Corps COSC. These functions are

- strengthen: to build strength by inducing stress, providing motivation, and supporting recovery
- mitigate: to control sources of stress that can be controlled
- identify: to identify Marines who are at increased risk of injury or illness as a result of stress exposure
- treat: to intervene early and get help to Marines in need
- reintegrate: to support Marines' reintegration into the unit after beginning treated for stress-related injury or illness.

We presented these items to the trainees on a list that also included "discipline" and asked them to identify the one item that is not a core leader function; 86 percent of respondents correctly identified "discipline" as the one item on the list that is not a core leader function.

Perceptions of Likely Reactions and Potential Changes as a Result of OSCAR

Table B.2 shows the respondents' perceptions of likely reactions from Marines and their leaders after returning to their units following their OSCAR training. Approximately three-quarters of all respondents agreed or strongly agreed that Marines would be willing to discuss their stress with them, and nearly all felt that their chains of command would support them in doing their jobs as OSCAR team members. At the same time, however, significant proportions of respondents also had perceptions that indicate potential risk for the OSCAR program, including agreeing or strongly agreeing that their chains of command might not believe that stress control is important (26 percent), that Marines who discuss their stress levels would be concerned about stigmatization (60 percent), and that Marines might be worried about confidentiality (38 percent).

Table B.3 shows respondents' beliefs about the extent to which OSCAR is likely to effect change in their units. Nearly all respondents felt that it was somewhat or very likely that Marines would be more willing to get help for stress when they need it; their units would be more ready for missions; Marines in their units would perform better; Marines in their units would feel more confident in themselves and their leaders; and Marines in their units would be healthier in body, mind, and spirit. However, only 61 percent of respondents felt that it was somewhat or very likely that Marines who need help for stress would spend less time away from their units getting that help. This represents a potential concern because one of the key goals of OSCAR is keeping Marines with their units and maintaining unit readiness.

Table B.2
Perceptions of Likely Reactions from Marines and Leaders After Returning to Their Units

Thinking About After You Return to Your Unit, to What Extent Do You Agree or Disagree with the Following Statements?	Response Indicates Negative Perception		Response Indicates Positive Perception	
	Neither Agree nor Disagree, Disagree, or Strongly Disagree		Agree or Strongly Agree	
	n	%	n	%
Marines will be willing to talk to me about their stress.	10	23.3	33	76.7
My chain of command will support me in doing my job as an OSCAR team member.	1	2.3	42	97.7
	Neither Agree nor Disagree, Agree or Strongly Agree		Disagree or Strongly Disagree	
My chain of command may not believe that stress control is important because tough and well-trained Marines don't have problems with stress.	11	25.6	32	74.4
Marines who talk to me about their stress will be worried that others in the unit will think less of them for it.	25	59.5	17	40.5
Marines who talk to me about their stress will be worried that what they tell me will not be confidential.	16	38.1	26	61.9

Table B.3
Beliefs About Potential Changes as a Result of OSCAR

How Likely Do You Think It Is That Each of the Following Will Happen Because of OSCAR?	Neither Unlikely nor Likely, Somewhat Unlikely, or Not Likely at All		Somewhat Likely or Very Likely	
	n	%	n	%
Marines will be more willing to get help for stress when they need it.	10	23.3	33	76.7
My unit will be more ready for its missions.	7	16.3	36	83.7
Marines who need help for stress will spend less time away from their units getting that help.	17	39.5	26	60.5
Marines in my unit will perform better.	14	32.6	29	67.4
Marines in my unit will feel more confident in themselves, each other, and their leaders.	12	27.9	31	72.1
Marines in my unit will be healthier in body, mind, and spirit.	11	25.6	32	74.4

Actions Respondents Reported They Would Take If Concerned About a Marine's Stress Level

We also included four vignettes with open-ended questions that allowed the respondents to describe how they would respond to Marines exhibiting different signs of stress. Two vignettes were administered before the training and two after. Two vignettes (one pretraining and one posttraining) depicted combat-related stress and behavior that should be a significant concern, such as a Marine openly stating the belief that he would be killed before returning home and who had altered speech patterns, or a Marine exhibiting inappropriate laughter, carelessness with weapons, and not seeming to care about himself or his fellow Marines. One of the vignettes, administered before the training, described a Marine displaying significant stress from non–combat-related causes. The remaining vignette discussed a Marine whose unit recently experienced casualties and who is a little quieter than usual but whose behavior does not represent a significant concern. The full text of the vignettes can be found in questions 4, 5, 10, and 11 in the survey shown at the end of this appendix.

Although the vignettes cannot be used to directly assess the impact of the OSCAR training in a quantitative manner, overall, the qualitative results (described in more detail below) suggest that responses to the posttraining vignettes were more likely to recommend actions in keeping with the principles taught in the OSCAR training and to use language consistent with that included in the training.

Vignettes Regarding Combat-Related Stress and More-Concerning Behavior

In one pretraining scenario, respondents were asked whether they were concerned about the stress level of a Marine nearing the end of a seven-month deployment to Afghanistan whose speech has changed (e.g., shaky voice, stuttering) and who expressed to others in his platoon a fear of being killed. They were also asked how they would respond to the situation. All respondents (100 percent) indicated that they were concerned about his level of stress. Most reported that they would talk to him to "listen to his thoughts," "find out what's going on," or "gauge how stressed he is." A few responded that they would provide mentorship and counseling regarding how to manage stress. Several respondents also indicated that they would refer him to the chaplain, medical officer, or battalion aid station. Of these, most noted that they would refer him after initially speaking with him to assess the situation, but some suggested they would immediately refer him to the chaplain, medical officer, battalion aid station, or "someone he feels comfortable talking to." One respondent indicated that he would have his platoon sergeant or commander "keep an eye on him" and "ensure they bring him in, talk to him, share their [perspective on] stress and make recommendations to me." Two respondents noted that they would pull him from combat duties or "rotate him off of being a driver."

In the posttraining scenario regarding combat-related stress and more-concerning behavior, respondents were asked whether a Marine who witnessed two serious casualties taken by his unit and subsequently did not seem to care about himself or his fellow Marines was in the orange zone; the majority (86 percent) felt that he was. When asked what they would do next, nearly all of the Marines responded that they would talk to him to "determine how severe his issues are," "to find out what he is dealing with," "get him to open up and stop trying to hide his stress," or "get him to express his feelings about the death of his friend." Posttraining, respondents tended to use terminology consistent with the principles described in the OSCAR training, such as "keep safe and calm, rest and recuperation, refer to medical and chaplain, mentor back to full duty." In addition, many respondents indicated that they would assess the situation and encourage or refer the Marine to get the care he needs.

Vignette Regarding Non–Combat-Related Stress

In this pretraining scenario, respondents were asked whether they were concerned about the stress level of a Marine who was increasingly aggressive, yet still performing his duties, after learning of his wife's infidelity. They were also asked what they would do in response to the situation. Almost all respondents (95 percent) indicated concern about his level of stress. Most reported that they would talk to him to "inform him that life will continue," "try to relate to him from personal experience," or "start spending more time with him to help him get through what he is dealing with." Others reported that they would refer him to a chaplain, to "counseling services," or to a medical officer. A few people suggested that they would find peers who were "having the same type of problems" to talk with him. Two respondents reported that they would inform the chain of command, and one respondent indicated that he would contact the Family Readiness Group to deal directly with the spouse.

However, a few respondents commented that they would take him off duty or "pull him off the road." In two cases, being taken off duty was framed as a punishment: "Inform him if his personal matters continue to show adverse potential that he will be given a 'break' from operations" and

> any violent outlash will be met with not an equal but an overwhelming reaction until he is controlled . . . once he has learned that violence towards others will only hurt himself . . . [and that] his pain is internal and cannot be attacked from the outside . . . he may return to operations.

These responses—given before the training began—are in contrast to the principles being emphasized in the OSCAR training (e.g., even the strongest Marines can be negatively affected by stress; Marines have a responsibility to address early signs of stress).

Vignette Regarding Less-Concerning Behavior

In this posttraining scenario, respondents were asked whether a Marine who was quieter than normal after his squad suffered two casualties during a recent firefight was in the orange zone; most (93 percent) did not feel that he was. When asked what they would do in response to the situation, almost all indicated that they would talk to him, to "explain to him that what he is feeling is normal," "help him deal with and express any feelings he may have from the firefight and deaths," and "offer a listening ear." Some suggested that they would employ his peers to talk with him. Three people suggested debriefing the entire platoon, with one suggesting an after-action review. Two reported that they would continue to monitor or observe him, with one suggesting relying on the chain of command to do so. Notably, several Marines used language reflective of the training, for example responding that the Marine was in the yellow zone, that they would "sit down with this Marine and get him back to the green zone," and "talk to him so he doesn't go into the orange zone." The described actions and the language used are consistent with the principles described in the OSCAR training.

Respondents' Assessment of the Training

In general, respondents rated the training highly. All or nearly all respondents agreed that, to some extent or a great extent, the trainers explained the content in easy-to-understand ways, listened carefully to their questions, and understood important information about how things worked in their units (see Table B.4). Conversely, only one respondent felt that the trainers had "talked down" to him. Nearly all respondents reported that their knowledge increased to some or a great extent as a result of the training, and most felt that they now had the skills to help Marines in need.

Table B.4
Respondents' Detailed Assessment of the Training

Measure	Not at All or Very Little		To Some Extent or to a Great Extent	
	n	%	*n*	%
To what extent did the trainers ...				
Explain things in a way that was easy to understand?	0	0.0	43	100.0
Listen carefully to questions that were asked?	0	0.0	43	100.0
Seem to know the important information about how things work in your unit?	2	4.7	41	95.4
Talk down to you?	42	97.7	1	2.3
Think about what you know about how to help a Marine who is experiencing stress:				
How much did your knowledge increase in this area because of the training?	3	7.1	39	92.9
To what extent do you feel that you now have the skills to help?	1	2.4	41	97.6

More globally, approximately two-thirds of respondents felt that the time spent at the training was about the right amount (see Table B.5). After the training, 47 percent of the respondents reported being very confident that they had the skills needed to do their jobs as OSCAR team members; all reported that they were at least somewhat confident. The six people who reported being only somewhat confident in their skills were evenly divided between officers and enlisted personnel.

On a 0-to-10 scale, where 10 represents the best possible training, nearly half of all respondents rated the training at an 8 or higher, with the remaining half rating the training between a 4 and a 7. In addition, 91 percent of respondents either agreed or strongly agreed with the statement "I have enough training or experience to do my job as an OSCAR team member well."

Respondents were also asked an open-ended question regarding changes they would like to see in the training. Four key themes emerged:

1. Several respondents asked for more real-world examples and stronger role-playing materials that better reflected reality. As one respondent noted, "Realistic scenarios with feedback from actual experience is what I found best." Another suggested that he would like to see "more experiences at actual combat being shared and what was learned from it." There were additional comments related specifically to the role playing, including suggestions that role playing should happen as each block of training content is completed and having senior and junior Marine Corps leaders role play together.

2. There were multiple requests to extend the training down to lower levels of Marines, with some requests to expand the training to all Marines. One respondent noted that "The attendee level should be changed to NCOs, being that [senior] NCOs and officers are rarely the first level of counsel [and] a certain degree of effectiveness is lost [if NCOs are not trained]." Another noted specifically that sergeants major would particularly benefit from attendance.

Table B.5
Respondents' Global Assessment of the Training

Measure	n	%
Was the time spent at training . . .		
A little too short or much too short	8	18.6
About right	28	65.1
A little too long or much too long	6	14.0
How confident are you that you now have the skills needed to do your job as an OSCAR team member?		
5 (very confident)	20	46.5
4	16	37.2
3 (somewhat confident)	6	14.0
2	0	0.0
1 (not at all confident)	0	0.0
Using any number from 0 to 10, where 0 is the worst training possible and 10 is the best training possible, what number would you use to rate this OSCAR training program?		
0–3	0	0.0
4–7	15	34.9
8–10	21	48.8

3. Three respondents felt that the material covered in the training reflected primarily basic leadership skills rather than specialized training. One of these people was an enlisted Marine; the other two were officers.

4. Finally, two areas were highlighted as content in need of greater attention during the training. The first of these is the need to pay more attention to the reintegration of Marines into the unit if they have been sent elsewhere for treatment, with one respondent noting "little time [was] spent on . . . reintegration to get rid of the stigma of seeking help." The second area reflects the respondents' concerns that they need more information regarding available services and how to access them for Marines who are in need, including one respondent who requested more information that would help him understand "what may be offered to [Marines] if they seek help." These two areas are the same as those highlighted in Table B.1 as potentially in need of greater emphasis during the training session.

Conclusions

In general, the training was well-regarded by the respondents, and they describe themselves as well-prepared to engage in their OSCAR roles upon return to their units.

Two areas indicate potential room for improvement in the contents of the training materials. First, in both the survey questions and in the open-ended question regarding what could be improved about the training, concerns were raised regarding knowledge and skills of the respondents for helping Marines reintegrate into their units after being treated somewhere else for stress. This likely relates in part to developing a skill set to help address the stigma of needing such treatment and in part to the need to have a plan and skill set in place to help coach Marines returning to their units in how to manage ongoing stress. Second, there were indications that, following the training, some respondents did not feel that they were aware of all of the resources available to help Marines experiencing high stress in theater and in garrison. This is an easier shortcoming to address because it requires the provision of factual information rather than imparting a new skill set.

In addition, the results of some of the posttraining survey questions indicate potential cause for concern, as some of the factors highlighted by respondents indicate threats to the likelihood of OSCAR's success. These include a significant proportion of respondents agreeing or strongly agreeing that their chain of command might not believe that stress control is important, that Marines who discuss their levels of stress control would have concerns about stigmatization, and that Marines would be concerned about confidentiality when discussing their stress levels with OSCAR team members. These factors are well known to the COSC program, which sponsors OSCAR, and OSCAR is in part an attempt to help bring about the cultural shift necessary in Marine Corps units to overcome these challenges.

Survey Instrument Administered at Training

We reproduce the survey instrument on the pages that follow.

7582212333

U.S. Marine Corps Operational Stress Control and Readiness (OSCAR) Program Evaluation Study

0 0 0

9437212334

As part of an evaluation of the OSCAR program, the RAND Corporation is inviting you to participate in an evaluation of the training you are attending. RAND is a non-profit research corporation, and this research study is being conducted on behalf of the Defense Centers of Excellence for Psychological Health and TBI and the Marine Combat and Operational Stress Control Program.

We are interested in finding out about your experience with being trained as an OSCAR team member. The goal of this part of the evaluation is to identify useful aspects of training as well as things that can be improved.

If you choose to participate in the training evaluation, you will complete a short questionnaire prior to the training, and an additional questionnaire immediately after the training. These questionnaires will ask about knowledge, how prepared you feel to be an OSCAR team member, challenges, and how likely you think it is that things will change back in your unit.

Your participation is completely voluntary and you have the option to stop at any time. All answers will be kept confidential. The questionnaires cannot be linked in any way to your name or other information that could be used to identify you. We will share only information about groups of people in our reports. Your individual answers will never be shared with anyone.

If you have any questions about this project, you may contact Robin Weinick at RAND, at 703-413-1100 x5151, or rweinick@rand.org.

Before the training starts, please complete only the information in questions 1 through 6 on pages 3 through 5. After the training ends, we will ask you to complete the remaining pages in this booklet. Please keep the whole booklet stapled together.

Thank you.

0 0 0

1214212339

Please complete this section before the training begins: Questions 1 through 6 on pages 3 through 5.

1. Are you being trained as an OSCAR:

☐ Extender

☐ Senior Mentor

☐ Peer Mentor

☐ Provider

☐ Other

☐ Don't know

2. What is your rank?

☐ E1-E3

☐ E4-E6

☐ E7-E9

☐ O1-O3

☐ O4-O6

☐ O7-O10

3. Have you previously participated in any training programs to help you recognize stress zones in your fellow Marines and/or intervene to restore their mental and spiritual well-being?

☐ Yes

☐ No

4736212331

4. LCpl Dan Daley is nearing the end of a seven-month deployment to Afghanistan, where he served as a driver in the Weapons Company of a ground combat unit. For the last few weeks, you have noticed that his speech has changed - his voice sounds shaky much of the time, and he has been stuttering a bit, something you never heard him do before. In addition, you have heard LCpl Daley tell others in his platoon that he is convinced he will be killed somehow before he can get on the plane to return home.

   a. Would you be concerned about the level of LCpl Daley's stress?

   ☐ Yes   ☐ No

   b. If LCpl Daley were in your unit, what would you do next?

   _____
   _____
   _____

5. A few weeks ago, shortly after returning from an uneventful patrol in Afghanistan, Cpl Smedley Butler was told by his wife that she didn't want to be married anymore, and was already seeing someone else. Since then, Cpl Butler has been constantly angry and has repeatedly lost his temper and screamed or thrown gear at subordinates and peers on his team. However, he has remained focused and effective when operating outside the wire, although he has been more aggressive than usual in his interactions with local civilians.

   a. Would you be concerned about the level of Cpl Butler's stress?

   ☐ Yes   ☐ No

   b. If Cpl Butler were in your unit, what would you do next?

   _____
   _____
   _____

0 0 0

4

6267212332

The next set of questions asks about how ready you feel, before the training, to do some of the things that OSCAR team members will be responsible for.

6. How prepared do you feel now to . . .

	Very unprepared	Somewhat unprepared	Somewhat prepared	Well prepared	Very well prepared
a. Know how to recognize stress zones that require help?	☐	☐	☐	☐	☐
b. Provide direct help to Marines who are in stress zones that place them at increased risk?	☐	☐	☐	☐	☐
c. Identify Marines in stress zones that place them at risk for either failing to perform their duties or developing long-term stress illnesses?	☐	☐	☐	☐	☐
d. Help restore the self-confidence of Marines who are recovering from stress injuries that briefly interfered with their job performance?	☐	☐	☐	☐	☐
e. Teach Marines in your unit how to monitor each others' stress zones and help each other reduce stress?	☐	☐	☐	☐	☐
f. Know which stress zones can be managed in the unit, and which require referral to a mental health professional?	☐	☐	☐	☐	☐
g. Help a Marine reintegrate into your unit after being treated somewhere else for stress?	☐	☐	☐	☐	☐
h. Know all the resources available to help Marines in a high stress zone, both in theater and at your home base?	☐	☐	☐	☐	☐
i. Advise and support your unit leadership to prevent, recognize, and take care of stress injuries?	☐	☐	☐	☐	☐

BEFORE the training begins:

PLEASE STOP HERE. Do not turn the page. Please place the questionnaire in the envelope it came in and keep it with you. At the end of the training, you will be asked to complete the rest of the questions in this package.

Thank you.

6873212335

Please start here only AFTER the training has ended. At that time, please complete the rest of the questions in this booklet, Questions 7 through 20 on Pages 6 through 11.

Now that the training is over, we would like to ask some questions that help us understand what you have learned about OSCAR.

7. To what extent do you agree or disagree with the following statements?

	Strongly disagree	Disagree	Neither agree nor disagree	Agree	Strongly agree
a. I understand my role as an OSCAR team member.	☐	☐	☐	☐	☐
b. I am confident that I can identify someone with an Orange Zone stress injury.	☐	☐	☐	☐	☐
c. I am confident that I know what to do when a Marine is in the Orange Zone.	☐	☐	☐	☐	☐

8. **Which of the following can be direct causes of Orange Zone stress injuries? Please mark all that apply:**

  ☐ Loss of others who are cared about

  ☐ Worries about money

  ☐ Inner conflict over morals and values

  ☐ Wear/tear accumulation of stress over time

  ☐ Arguments with a spouse

  ☐ Immediate threat to your own life

  ☐ Not getting along with other Marines in your unit

9. **Which of the following is NOT a core leader function for Combat Operational Stress Control? Please mark only one:**

  ☐ Strengthen

  ☐ Mitigate

  ☐ Identify

  ☐ Discipline

  ☐ Treat

  ☐ Reintegrate

0 0 0

1999212339

10. PFC Lewis Puller just returned to the FOB from his first firefight in Afghanistan, during which two serious casualties were taken by his unit. One of the Marines killed in that firefight was another PFC who joined the unit from the School of Infantry at the same time as PFC Puller. Since returning, PFC Puller has been laughing at inappropriate times, even during briefings and other serious conversations, almost as though he can't stop. In addition, he has been sloppy with his gear and uniform, and careless with his weapon, not seeming to care about himself or his fellow Marines.

    a. Is PFC Puller in the Orange Zone?

        ☐ Yes   ☐ No

    b. If PFC Puller were in your unit, what would you do next?

_____

_____

_____

11. LCpl Jose Ruiz was also a member of the squad that suffered two casualties during a recent firefight in Afghanistan. Since returning from that patrol, LCpl Ruiz has seemed a little quieter than usual, and keeping to himself a little more, but has been able to carry out all his normal duties without difficulty, and has otherwise seemed like his normal self.

    a. Is LCpl Ruiz in the Orange Zone?

        ☐ Yes   ☐ No

    b. If LCpl Ruiz were in your unit, what would you do next?

_____

_____

_____

0   0   0

7

0699212335

The next set of questions asks about how ready you feel to do some of the things that OSCAR team members will be responsible for. Please think about how you feel now compared to how you felt before the OSCAR training started.

12. Compared to before your OSCAR training, how prepared do you feel to . . .

	Less prepared	About the same	Somewhat more prepared	Much more prepared
a. Know how to recognize stress zones that require help?	☐	☐	☐	☐
b. Provide direct help to Marines who are in stress zones that place them at increased risk?	☐	☐	☐	☐
c. Identify Marines in stress zones that place them at risk for either failing to perform their duties or developing long-term stress illnesses?	☐	☐	☐	☐
d. Help restore the self-confidence of Marines who are recovering from stress injuries that briefly interfered with their job performance?	☐	☐	☐	☐
e. Teach Marines in your unit how to monitor each others' stress zones and help each other reduce stress?	☐	☐	☐	☐
f. Know which stress zones can be managed in the unit, and which require referral to a mental health professional?	☐	☐	☐	☐
g. Help a Marine reintegrate into your unit after being treated somewhere else for stress?	☐	☐	☐	☐
h. Know all the resources available to help Marines in a high stress zone, both in theater and at your home base?	☐	☐	☐	☐
i. Advise and support your unit leadership to prevent, recognize, and take care of stress injuries?	☐	☐	☐	☐
j. Support your unit leadership in helping Marines deal with stress?	☐	☐	☐	☐

0 0 0

6784212336

Next, we would like to know what you think about what things will be like after you return to your unit.

13. Thinking about after you return to your unit, to what extent to you agree or disagree with the following statements?

	Strongly disagree	Disagree	Neither agree nor disagree	Agree	Strongly agree
a. I have enough training or experience to do my job as an OSCAR team member well.	☐	☐	☐	☐	☐
b. Marines will be willing to talk to me about their stress.	☐	☐	☐	☐	☐
c. My chain of command will support me in doing my job as an OSCAR team member.	☐	☐	☐	☐	☐
d. My chain of command may not believe that stress control is important because tough and well-trained Marines don't have problems with stress.	☐	☐	☐	☐	☐
e. Marines who talk to me about their stress will be worried that others in the unit will think less of them for it.	☐	☐	☐	☐	☐
f. Marines who talk to me about their stress will be worried that what they tell me will not be confidential.	☐	☐	☐	☐	☐

4935212332

Now we would like to know your thoughts on what might happen now that the Marines have the OSCAR program.

14. How likely do you think it is that each of the following will happen because of OSCAR?

	Not likely at all	Somewhat unlikely	Neither unlikely nor likely	Somewhat likely	Very likely
a. Marines will be more willing to get help for stress when they need it.	☐	☐	☐	☐	☐
b. My unit will be more ready for its missions.	☐	☐	☐	☐	☐
c. Marines who need help for stress will spend less time away from their units getting that help.	☐	☐	☐	☐	☐
d. Marines in my unit will perform better.	☐	☐	☐	☐	☐
e. Marines in my unit will feel more confident in themselves, each other, and their leaders.	☐	☐	☐	☐	☐
f. Marines in my unit will be healthier in body, mind, and spirit.	☐	☐	☐	☐	☐

Finally, we would like to ask some questions about the training you just completed.

15. To what extent did the trainers . . .

	Not at all	Very little	To some extent	To a great extent
a. Explain things in a way that was easy to understand?	☐	☐	☐	☐
b. Listen carefully to questions that were asked?	☐	☐	☐	☐
c. Seem to know the important information about how things work in your unit?	☐	☐	☐	☐
d. Talk down to you?	☐	☐	☐	☐

0 0 0

9217212330

16. Think about what you know about how to help a Marine who is experiencing stress.

	Not at all	Very little	To some extent	To a great extent
a. How much did your knowledge increase in this area because of the training?	☐	☐	☐	☐
b. To what extent do you feel that you now have the skills to help?	☐	☐	☐	☐

17. Was the time spent at training . . .

Much too short	A little too short	About right	A little too long	Much too long
☐	☐	☐	☐	☐

18. How confident are you that you now have the skills needed to do your job as an OSCAR team member?

Not at all confident 1	2	Somewhat confident 3	4	Very confident 5
☐	☐	☐	☐	☐

19. Using any number from 0 to 10, where 0 is the worst training possible and 10 is the best training possible, what number would you use to rate this OSCAR training program?

0 ☐ Worst training possible
1 ☐
2 ☐
3 ☐
4 ☐
5 ☐
6 ☐
7 ☐
8 ☐
9 ☐
10 ☐ Best training possible

20. What should be changed about the training you just completed?

_____
_____
_____
_____

3315212333

**Please place this questionnaire in the envelope,
seal the envelope,
and return the envelope to the RAND staff members who are here today.**

Thank you very much for your help.

0   0   0

Detailed Description of Individual Marine Survey Methods

This appendix contains a detailed description of the sampling, procedures, measures, and statistical analysis for the individual Marine survey component of the OSCAR evaluation.

Sampling

We followed a two-stage sampling procedure that consisted of (1) sampling eligible battalions and then (2) sampling companies from each of the battalions sampled. In the first stage, our contacts in the COSC office identified battalions that met our eligibility criteria, which consisted of active-duty or reserve units preparing for a combat deployment to Iraq or Afghanistan in 2010 or 2011. We sampled six battalions scheduled to undergo OSCAR training prior to deployment, including four infantry battalions and two service-support battalions (i.e., combat logistics and engineering support battalions) and two battalions that were not scheduled to receive OSCAR training prior to deployment,[1] both of which were service-support battalions. Two of the OSCAR-trained battalions and both of the control battalions were augmented by Marines from other battalions prior to deployment to form larger composite units, each of which functioned as a single unit during deployment. Collectively, these four composite battalions included Marines from 12 "parent" battalions. Altogether, the eight battalions sampled included Marines from 16 "parent" battalions.

In the second stage of sampling, companies were sampled from within each of the battalions sampled in the first stage. Given variability in the organization of battalions and their ability to accommodate our requests for survey coordination, the procedure for sampling companies varied across battalions, and thus the number of Marines per sampled battalion varied as well. We sampled between three and five companies from each of the four infantry battalions in the OSCAR-trained group. Companies were randomly sampled from each of the first two infantry battalions sampled. Because random sampling proved very logistically challenging to implement, we sampled all available companies from the two remaining infantry battalions. From both of the composite service-support battalions in the OSCAR-trained group, we sampled only a single company because this recruitment fully met our targeted sample size for the OSCAR-trained group. We attempted to recruit all available companies from both of

---

[1] Because of a MARADMIN released from HQMC in October 2011 that mandated dissemination of OSCAR to all battalions in the USMC by January 31, 2012, we had difficulty identifying battalions that had not received OSCAR training to enroll in the control group and thus reaching our targeted sample size for the control group. Therefore, our sample size for the control group is roughly half of that for the intervention group.

the composite service-support battalions in the control group. Figure C.1 depicts the two-stage sampling strategy.

All Marines of rank O6 (colonel) or lower within each company were sampled for T1 survey participation. However, to be included in this analysis,[2] Marines also had to have deployed to Iraq or Afghanistan after the T1 survey as expected. A total of 2,975 Marines were known to have had the opportunity to enroll in the study.[3] Of these Marines, 2,620 Marines completed the T1 survey,[4] of which 96.3 percent (*n* = 2,523) were eligible for inclusion in this analysis. Among the 2,523 Marines, 1,631 were in battalions that subsequently received OSCAR training, and 892 were in battalions that did not receive OSCAR training. We computed the response rate for the T1 survey as the number of study-eligible survey completers (2,523) divided by the number of Marines (completers and decliners) who were eligible for inclusion in the analysis, which equals 2,865 (96.3 percent of 2,975).[5] Therefore, the response rate for the T1 survey was 88.1 percent (2,523 ÷ 2,865).

Of the 2,523 eligible Marines who completed the T1 survey, 51.8 percent also completed the T2 survey, resulting in a final sample size of 1,307. The final sample was composed

Figure C.1
OSCAR Individual Marine Survey Study Design

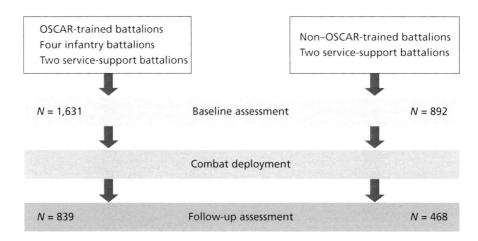

SOURCE: Department of Veterans Affairs and DoD, 2009.
RAND RR562-C.1

---

[2]   A secondary analysis of T1 survey data was conducted, and the findings and recommendations from this analysis are described in a separate report (Farmer et al., 2014). The secondary analysis made use of available data on all T1 survey respondents (*N* = 2,620), not just those who were eligible for inclusion in this analysis to evaluate OSCAR.

[3]   This number underestimates the number of Marines who could have participated in the study. There might have been other Marines in the units targeted for the survey who were eligible to participate and passively refused by not returning their survey or returning it blank without explicitly indicating their refusal to participate on the survey. In the absence of a returned survey with a marking on it to acknowledge the decision to participate (or not), we do not know whether the Marine had the opportunity to participate in the survey.

[4]   A total of 355 Marines explicitly declined to participate in the T1 survey.

[5]   We were unable to determine the eligibility of the 355 Marines who declined to participate in the survey (i.e., whether they deployed to Iraq or Afghanistan). In calculating the denominator for the response rate, we assume that the proportion of eligible Marines among those who declined is the same as the proportion of eligible Marines among the survey completers; i.e., 96.3 percent of the Marines who declined to participate would have been eligible for inclusion in the analysis.

of 839 Marines in OSCAR-trained battalions and 468 Marines in non–OSCAR-trained battalions.

Procedures

Data collection took place between March 2010 and October 2012. For respondents in OSCAR-trained battalions, to obtain a baseline assessment of T2 outcomes of interest, T1 surveys were almost always administered prior to the battalion's OSCAR training.[6] The amount of time between the dates of the T1 survey administration and deployment varied across battalions, with an average (mean) of 61.1 days (SD = 46.8 days) between the T1 survey and the date of deployment (minimum: 13 days; maximum: 6.5 months).

Once a subset of companies in the battalion to target for recruitment had been identified, we coordinated with a POC in the unit to determine a date and time for the T1 survey when the majority of the Marines would be available. The unit POC then arranged for the Marines to come to the survey administration site at the agreed-upon date and time. At the beginning of the survey administration, a survey administrator would read the HSPC-approved oral consent script describing the study's purpose and relevant information about human subjects' research protections (e.g., the voluntary nature of participation, protection of confidentiality of survey responses). After the script was read, the Marines were asked to decide whether to participate and to indicate their decision on the front page of the survey. Each Marine, regardless of his or her decision to participate, was asked to return the survey to the survey administrator in a blank envelope provided with the survey after finishing it.

Given that military populations are accustomed to following orders and the potential for prospective survey participants to misconstrue the survey as mandatory, several measures were taken to avert this misperception and mitigate pressure to participate in the study. Survey arrangements were coordinated with a unit POC who was not in the chain of command, typically a Marine in the operations section (S-3). Unit commands were not permitted to be in the room at the time of survey administration. Survey administrators were required to be outside the chain of command and typically included members of the RAND team, COSC personnel, or the unit chaplain or RP. Prior to the survey administration, survey administrators who were not RAND staff were required to read survey administration instructions that delineated their role in protecting the confidentiality of individual Marines' decisions regarding participation and individual survey responses and to affirm in writing (or via email) their understanding and agreement to abide by the prescribed survey procedures.

We also took care to communicate to prospective participants the nature and extent of the protections applied to maintain the confidentiality of individual survey responses and the purpose for which survey data were being collected. Similar questionnaires that cover sensitive topics such as mental health and alcohol use, e.g., the Postdeployment Health Assessment (PDHA), are routinely used in the military to inform decisions regarding screening, referral, and treatment of mental health and substance use problems and included in the person's military record. To distinguish our survey from similar questionnaires used in the military,

---

[6]   In one battalion, it was not possible to administer the T1 survey before OSCAR training had been conducted. However, the survey was administered before the unit underwent combat simulation training and thus prior to the unit's exposure to stress of a nature similar to that experienced in combat and that which OSCAR is principally designed to address.

we emphasized in the oral consent script and survey instructions that the participant's individual responses to this survey would be used only for research, would never be shared with anyone outside the RAND research team, and would never be tied to the participant's military record in any way. This clarification was important both from a human subjects' protection standpoint and from a data quality standpoint given research indicating that mental health problems tend to be underestimated when based on data collected without anonymity, e.g., the PDHA (Warner et al., 2011).

We aimed to administer the T2 survey in a group setting on base approximately two to three months after redeployment from Iraq or Afghanistan. This length of time was intended to permit the passage of enough time after redeployment for Marines' perceptions of their deployment experiences to stabilize while still surveying the Marines when their deployment experiences would be relatively recent and easily recalled. However, primarily because of the units' scheduling constraints, the length of time between the dates of the unit's redeployment and the T2 survey varied considerably, such that an average of 92.2 days (SD = 3.4 months) lapsed between them (minimum: four days; maximum: 17.5 months).

Of the 2,523 eligible Marines who completed the T1 survey, 51.8 percent also completed the T2 survey, resulting in a final sample size of 1,307. Only a small percentage of T1 survey completers explicitly refused to complete the T2 survey (n = 194, 7.7 percent). Rather, most Marines who did not complete the T2 survey simply could not be located after redeployment. Based on information conveyed informally by our POCs in the units we surveyed, the primary causes of attrition, i.e., loss of study participants between the T1 and T2 surveys, seem to have been types of transitions that often occur soon after redeployment—namely, a PCS or the EAS. Marines who had PCS'ed or EAS'ed soon after redeployment were not available on base to complete the T2 survey when it was administered to their units. When a Marine was not present at the on-base T2 survey administration, we mailed the T2 survey to his or her home address in an effort to maximize the study retention rate. A total of 717 T1 survey respondents unavailable for the on-base T2 survey administration were mailed surveys, and only 61 (8.5 percent) returned a completed survey. The completion of some T2 surveys by mail further increased the length of time between redeployment and the T2 survey.

To assess the impact of attrition on the final sample composition, we conducted cluster-adjusted Wald chi-square tests of significance to compare the T2 survey completers (n = 1,307) and noncompleters (n = 1,216) on all of the sociodemographic and service history characteristics and baseline levels of the outcomes of interest measured in the T1 survey (see Table 3.1 in Chapter Three for a list of outcomes measured in the T1 survey). The two groups differed significantly only on parental status and deployment history.[7] Marines who did not complete the T2 survey were more likely to have children and to have deployed previously to Iraq or Afghanistan at least once.

---

[7]   Tests of significance and descriptive statistics on the variables on which differences were found were as follows: The two groups differed significantly only on parental status (Wald chi-square = 7.58, p = 0.01) and deployment history (Wald chi-square = 5.79, p = 0.03). Marines who did not complete the T2 survey were more likely to have one child or more (noncompleters: 24.0 percent parents; completers: 19.8 percent parents) and to have deployed previously to Iraq or Afghanistan at least once (noncompleters: 50.4 percent previously deployed; completers: 34.1 percent previously deployed).

Measures

In this section, we describe the measures used in the individual Marine survey in detail, including their psychometric properties and how they were scored for inclusion in the main analysis of OSCAR's impact. Measures are grouped into three major categories: covariates, proximal outcomes, and distal outcomes.

Before describing the measures, we briefly define some of the terms used in reference to their psychometric properties. *Reliability* refers to consistency of measurement. Although reliability has multiple facets (e.g., test–retest reliability, alternate-forms reliability), the primary facet of reliability that we report here is the internal consistency of the measures, or how well participants' responses to items in a measure cohere. That is, do respondents similarly endorse items that tap similar content? We report Cronbach's alpha, an index of internal consistency that ranges from 0 to 1.00, with higher scores indicating higher internal consistency. In general, a Cronbach's alpha below 0.70 is considered unacceptable. We also refer to the validity of a measure, which is the extent to which the measure captures the construct it is intended to measure. Specific types of validity reported here are convergent validity, which is the extent to which scores on a measure converge or correlate positively with scores on other measures of similar constructs; criterion-related validity, which is the extent to which scores on a measure predict a criterion (i.e., outcome) that they would be expected to predict; and discriminant validity, which is the extent to which a measure effectively discriminates between different groups as expected.

Two types of psychometric properties that are used to describe the performance of measures that have been developed to screen for a particular condition, such as alcohol dependence, are sensitivity and specificity. *Sensitivity* refers to the proportion of people who have the condition (e.g., alcohol dependence) according to a gold-standard assessment, such as a structured clinical interview, and are correctly identified by the screener (e.g., AUDIT-C) as having the condition (e.g., 54 percent of people who met diagnostic criteria for alcohol dependence based on a structured clinical interview in a previous study by Dawson et al. [2005] were correctly classified as having alcohol dependence using a cutoff score of 8 or higher on the AUDIT-C). *Specificity*, in contrast, refers to the proportion of people who do not have the condition according to a gold-standard assessment and are correctly identified as not having the condition by the screener (e.g., 94 percent of people who did not meet criteria for alcohol dependence based on a structured clinical interview were correctly classified as not having alcohol dependence based on a score of less than 8 on the AUDIT-C) (Dawson et al., 2005).

Covariates
Sociodemographic and Service History Characteristics
In the T1 survey, each respondent was asked to report his or her rank, age, ethnicity, race, marital status, number of children, and the number of previous deployments to Iraq or Afghanistan since 2001.[8] Each respondent was also asked how many times he or she had attended a stress class prior to or since joining his or her current unit on a scale that ranged from "never" to "almost all of the time." Other service history characteristics determined from administrative data for inclusion as covariates in regression models were the number of days between the

---

[8]   Sex was not assessed on the survey because of concerns that this would greatly increase the risk of identifiability of female survey respondents because women constitute a very small proportion of Marines.

T1 survey administration and the date of deployment and the number of days between the T2 survey administration and the date of redeployment.

Lifetime History of Potentially Traumatic Events

In the T1 survey, the LEC (Gray et al., 2004) was used to assess direct exposure to 17 different types of stressful events, such as a natural disaster; physical assault; assault with a weapon; combat or exposure to a war zone; life-threatening illness or injury; or serious injury, harm, or death the respondent caused to someone else. Past research has documented the adequacy of the LEC's temporal stability and convergent validity with another established measure of trauma exposure (Gray et al., 2004). Importantly, the convergent validity of the LEC has also been demonstrated in a sample of combat veterans via its associations with measures of psychological distress and PTSD symptoms (Gray et al., 2004).

For regression models, we created a series of indicators to represent different theoretically meaningful categories of types of events directly experienced, in which indicators were coded 1 if the respondent reported any one of the events subsumed under the category and 0 if the respondent did not report any of the events in the category. Seven broad categories were created: accidents and disasters (natural disaster, fire or explosion, motor vehicle accident, other serious accident, or exposure to toxic substance); nonsexual assault (physical assault, assault with a weapon, combat, or captivity); sexual assault or other unwanted sexual experience; witnessing violent death or experienced the sudden, unexpected death of a loved one; experiencing a life-threatening illness or injury; causing serious injury or death of another; and experiencing another type of very stressful event.

Combat Experiences During Deployment

The frequency with which respondents had various stereotypical combat experiences during their most recent deployments was assessed in the T2 survey with ten items from the DRRI Combat Experiences subscale (King et al., 2006). Example items include "I was in a vehicle that was under fire" and "My unit engaged in battle in which it suffered casualties." Respondents indicated the frequency of each experience on a 0 (never) to 4 (daily or almost daily) scale. The Combat Experiences subscale has evidenced criterion-related validity through significant associations with mental health measures in past research (King et al., 2006; Vogt et al., 2008). Discriminant validity is indicated by significantly higher scores on this subscale observed among combat-support military personnel than those for service-support personnel, who would be expected to have less exposure to combat experiences because of their role in the military (Vogt et al., 2008). In the current study, composite scores on this measure were computed by summing the ratings of the frequency of the ten events assessed. Possible scores range from 0 to 40, with higher scores indicating more-frequent exposure to more types of combat experiences.

Peritraumatic Distress

The 15-item PBQ-SR (Nash, Goldwasser, et al., 2009) was administered in the T2 survey to assess peritraumatic distress and dissociation at the time of the respondent's most stressful experience during his or her most recent deployment. Each item was assessed on a scale ranging from 1 (not at all true) to 5 (completely true). Item responses were summed to generate a total scale score on which the range of possible scores is 15 to 75. Support for the PBQ-SR's reliability and validity comes from a pilot study conducted with 145 active-duty service members and veterans with histories of combat exposure in Iraq or Afghanistan. The PBQ-SR demonstrated excellent internal consistency (Cronbach's alpha = 0.90); convergent validity through its significant, positive correlation with the Clinician-Administered PTSD Scale (r = 0.66); and discriminant validity via its negative correlation with the SF-36 Physical Functioning scale (Nash, Goldwasser, et al., 2009). In the current study, internal consistency was also excellent (Cronbach's alpha = 0.90).

Deployment Environment

Irritations and discomfort experienced during the Marine's most recent deployment were assessed in the T2 survey with 20 items from the DRRI Difficulty Living and Working Environment subscale (King et al., 2006). Example items include "I had to deal with annoying animals, insects, or plants during my deployment" and "The food I had to eat was of very poor quality." Respondents indicated the frequency of each experience on a 1 (almost none of the time) to 5 (almost all of the time). Item responses were summed to generate a total scale score on which possible scores ranged from 20 to 100. This scale has evidenced excellent internal consistency reliability in previous research (Cronbach's alpha = 0.87, 0.89) (King et al., 2006). Convergent validity of this subscale is suggested by its significant, positive correlations with measures of PTSD, depression, and anxiety (King et al., 2006). In the current study, internal consistency was high (Cronbach's alpha = 0.84).

Proximal Outcomes
Attitudes Toward Stress Response and Recovery

In both the T1 and T2 surveys, we assessed stress-related perceptions and attitudes, including respondents' self-perceived readiness; self-efficacy to handle their own stress and to help peers handle their own stress; perceived efficacy of their peers and leaders to resolve their own stress problems and help respondents resolve their own stress problems; beliefs about the extent to which the responsibility to handle stress problems is shared by all Marines; and perceived stigmatization of and support for seeking help for stress problems at the level of the respondent's peers, leaders, unit, and the Marine Corps overall. Respondents indicated the extent to which they agreed with items on a scale of 1 to 5.

We developed two scales from these items: (1) a 13-item scale of positive expectancies toward coping with and recovering from stress and (2) a ten-item scale of perceived stigmatization of stress and seeking help for stress problems. All items were scored in a positive direction to indicate healthier perceptions and attitudes related to stress response and recovery prior to computing the mean of item ratings to obtain a composite scale score. Possible scores on both of the scales range from 1 to 5. Higher scores connote more-positive (i.e., healthier) perceptions and attitudes toward stress response and recovery. Both of the scales evidenced high internal consistency at both time points (range of Cronbach's alpha estimates = 0.82–0.85). Additional information on the development of these scales is available in another report based on data collected for this evaluation (Farmer et al., 2014).

Use of Social Resources for Stress

Respondents were asked about their use of different types of social resources in response to stress problems. Survey items assessed respondents' reports both of their own reliance on each of several resources for stress and of recommendation of the same resources to fellow Marines for help with stress. Possible resources included the following: oneself, fellow Marine, leader, corpsman, chaplain, and unit medical officer.

Separate indicators were created for seeking help from and recommending to fellow Marines each of these types of resources, e.g., seeking help for one's own stress from a peer was one indicator. Indicators were coded 1 to indicate that the respondent reported having sought help from (or recommended) the resource or 0 if the respondent had not. A similar set of indicators was created for whether the respondent had recommended each type of resource to a fellow Marine for help with stress problems. Two additional indicators were created for (1) whether the respondent had sought help from any of the types of resources and (2) whether the respondent had recommended any of the types of resources to a fellow Marine for help with stress.

Unit Support

Marines' perceptions of the supportiveness of the military in general, unit leaders, and other unit members were assessed in the T1 and T2 surveys with the 12-item Deployment Social Support subscale of the DRRI (King et al., 2006). Example items include "My unit is like family to me" and "I am supported by the Marine Corps." Each item was rated on a scale ranging from 1 (strongly disagree) to 5 (strongly agree). Composite scale scores were computed as the mean of item ratings. This scale has evidenced excellent internal consistency reliability in previous research (Cronbach's alpha = 0.91, 0.94) (King et al., 2006). The concurrent validity of this scale is supported by significant, negative correlations with PTSD, depression, and anxiety (King et al., 2006). In the current study, internal consistency was excellent in the T1 survey (Cronbach's alpha = 0.93) and T2 survey (Cronbach's alpha = 0.94).

Distal Outcomes

Current Stress

Each respondent was asked to rate his or her current level of stress on the COSC (e.g. green, yellow, orange, or red). This variable was dichotomized such that Marines who endorsed the orange or red zones were combined into one category, and Marines who endorsed the green or yellow zones were combined into another category.

Posttraumatic Stress Disorder

In the T1 survey, symptoms of PTSD were assessed with a modified version of the PCL-C (Ruggiero et al., 2003), in which respondents were asked to indicate on a five-point scale the extent to which they had experienced each of 17 symptoms "in your lifetime" as opposed to the standard time frame of "past 30 days." This was used as a proxy for lifetime self-reported PTSD, for which no current self-report measure exists. In psychometric research, the standard PCL-C has evidenced high internal consistency reliability (Cronbach's alpha = 0.94), convergent validity via its correlations with other well-established measures of PTSD (i.e., the Impact of Event Scale and Mississippi Scale for PTSD), and discriminant validity via its stronger correlations with PTSD-specific symptom measures relative to its correlations with measures of general psychopathology (Ruggiero et al., 2003). Factor loadings of the items on the PCL-C have been shown to be invariant across U.S. military personnel with and without a history of deployment in the past year (Mansfield et al., 2010). A composite scale score was computed by summing item responses. Possible scale scores range from 17 to 85, with higher scores indicating greater severity of PTSD symptoms experienced over the course of one's lifetime. Internal consistency for item responses in the T1 survey was excellent (Cronbach's alpha = 0.95).

In the T2 survey, respondents completed the PCL-C, but the standard time frame of past month for reporting symptoms was used. Internal consistency for the PCL-C in the T2 survey was excellent (Cronbach's alpha = 0.96). Probable diagnoses of current PTSD were derived based on the cluster scoring method (Weathers, Litz, et al., 1993). In particular, symptoms were counted as present if respondents indicated that they had been "moderately (3)" bothered by the symptom. Symptoms were then scored according to the *Diagnostic and Statistical Manual of Mental Disorders*, fourth edition (DSM-IV) definition. This scoring has been shown to have high specificity and sensitivity, 0.92 and 1.00, respectively (see Brewin, 2005, for a review of different scoring methods).

Depression

In the T1 survey, the PHQ-2 (Kroenke, Strine, et al., 2009) was used to screen for MDD. This two-item screener assesses the frequency with which depressed mood and anhedonia, i.e., the inability to derive pleasure from activities once enjoyed, were experienced in the past two weeks on a four-point (0–3) scale. In the current study, the time frame over which symptoms were assessed was the past month instead of the past two weeks. Included as a covariate in analyses, the PHQ-2 was scored continuously by summing item responses to the two questions to generate a total scale score that ranges from 0 to 6, with higher scores indicating more-frequent depressed mood and anhedonia.

In the T2 survey, we used the PHQ-8 (Kroenke, Spitzer, and Williams, 2001; Löwe et al., 2004) to assess probable MDD. The PHQ-8 is keyed to the DSM-IV criteria for MDD, excluding the suicide item. Like they are for the PHQ-2, respondents are asked to report the frequency with which they experienced each symptom in the past two weeks on a four-point (0–3) scale. We determined probable MDD by summing the item responses and counting respondents with scores of 10 or greater as positive for probable MDD. This cutpoint has been shown to have excellent specificity (0.92) and sensitivity (0.99) in the detection of clinical diagnoses (Kroenke, Spitzer, and Williams, 2001).

High-Risk Alcohol Use

The AUDIT-C (Bush et al., 1998) was used to screen for high-risk alcohol use in both the T1 and T2 surveys. This is a three-item measure that queries respondents about their frequency and quantity of alcohol consumption in the past year. Possible scores range from 0 to 12, and the higher the score, the more likely it is that the respondent's drinking is affecting his or her health and safety. Based on the Department of Veterans Affairs/DoD guidelines for management of substance use disorders, which recommend a referral to specialty care for substance use disorders for anyone with a score of 8 or higher on the AUDIT-C (Department of Veterans Affairs and Department of Defense, 2009), we used a cutoff score of 8 or higher to categorize participants' self-reported drinking behavior as high risk. This cut score has been shown to have a sensitivity of 0.54 and specificity of 0.94 in the detection of alcohol dependence in previous research (Dawson et al., 2005). Internal consistency for the AUDIT-C was good at both time points (T1 survey: Cronbach's alpha = 0.87; T2 survey: Cronbach's alpha = 0.86).

General Health

General health was assessed at both time points with a single item from the SF-12 (Ware, Kosinski, and Keller, 1996) asking respondents to rate their general health on a scale ranging from 1 (excellent) to 5 (poor). We scored this measure based on the recommendations of Hays, Sherbourne, and Mazel (1993). Subscale scores range from 0 to 100, with higher scores indicating better health. The reliability and validity of the SF-12 have been documented in past research (Ware, Kosinski, and Keller, 1996).

Occupational Impairment

Occupational impairment was assessed at both time points with a five-item scale from the HPQ (Kessler et al., 2003). Items assess the frequency of impairment in work performance in the past four weeks in the areas of productivity, carefulness, quality of work produced, and concentration. One item assesses the extent to which the respondent's work performance has been limited by health problems. Items are rated on a five-point scale ranging from 1 (none of the time) to 5 (all of the time) and averaged to compute a composite scale score. In the current study, internal consistency was excellent at both time points (T1 survey: Cronbach's alpha = 0.88; T2 survey: Cronbach's alpha = 0.90).

Statistical Analysis

To evaluate OSCAR's impact on the outcomes of interest, we conducted difference-in-differences analyses in which we compared Marines in the OSCAR-trained and control battalions on pre- to postdeployment differences in key outcomes. Analyses included a series of multivariate logistic regression models in which we estimated the impact of OSCAR on changes over time in key outcomes while adjusting for baseline characteristics and deployment experiences that could potentially confound OSCAR's effects. Models were estimated in SAS 9.2 PROC SURVEYLOGISTIC. Membership in OSCAR-trained battalions or control battalions was operationalized analytically as a dichotomous predictor (1 = intervention or OSCAR-trained battalions; 0 = control or non–OSCAR-trained battalions). Changes in continuous outcomes were operationalized analytically by dichotomizing outcomes into categories of "improved" versus "did not change" or "declined" between the T1 and T2 surveys. Changes in categorical outcomes were operationalized analytically by including baseline levels of the categorical outcome in the prediction of postdeployment levels of the categorical outcome, i.e., estimating residualized change models. To simplify the interpretation of the results, the method of recycled predictions was used to translate the model results into the predicted prevalence of each outcome with and without OSCAR training (Graubard and Korn, 1999; Setodji et al., 2012).

All statistical analyses of OSCAR's impact on outcomes were weighted to represent the average treatment effects among the Marines in OSCAR-trained battalions and adjusted for the clustering of participants within battalions.[9] Because the study design was quasi-experimental, i.e., battalions received OSCAR training at the discretion of Marine Corps leadership rather than having an equal chance of receiving OSCAR as the result of random assignment,[10] and Marines in the OSCAR-trained and control battalions differed on several potentially confounding baseline characteristics and deployment experiences, it was necessary to adjust sta-

---

[9] We adjusted for clustering effects at the level of the 16 "parent" battalions, rather than the eight "composite" battalions described in the "Sampling" section of Chapter Three, because of the greater cohesion and thus commonality of outcomes that typically characterize smaller groups.

[10] At the inception of data collection in March 2010, infantry units received priority for OSCAR training over service-support units, such as combat logistics and engineering support battalions.

tistically for these group differences. We adjusted for these differences with a doubly robust method that included propensity score weighting and the inclusion of baseline characteristics and deployment experiences as predictors in the model. Created in the Generalized Boosted Regression Models package in R, propensity scores were calculated in logistic regression models with all baseline and deployment-related variables entered as predictors. All of the covariates and baseline levels of the outcomes listed in Table 3.1 in Chapter Three were included as predictors in the models estimated to create propensity score weights and as covariates in the multivariate regression models estimating OSCAR's impact on outcomes. However, because the type of battalion (infantry versus service support) was so highly confounded with treatment group (OSCAR-trained versus control battalion), we were unable to include it as a predictor in models to create propensity scores or in multivariate regression models to estimate OSCAR's impact on outcomes. In an attempt to disentangle OSCAR's effects from that of battalion type, we performed a sensitivity analysis to examine OSCAR's impact on outcomes among the subset of Marines in service-support battalions and determine whether the pattern of findings obtained in the full sample could be replicated. That is, we estimated a series of multivariate models to compare the Marines in the OSCAR-trained service-support battalions ($n = 90$) and those in the non–OSCAR-trained service-support battalions ($n = 468$). A separate set of propensity weights was created for this analysis.

Although the final sample size was 1,307, the total number of cases included in multivariate models estimated without adjustment for missing data ranged from 972 to 1,063 across outcomes. To assess the extent to which the loss of participants who had missing data on one or more variables included in multivariate models might have biased the parameter estimates, we conducted a sensitivity analysis in which we estimated a series of multivariate models with multiple imputation of missing data, a strategy recommended for handling missing data under the assumption that data are missing at random (Schafer and Graham, 2002). We then compared the results for the models with and without multiple imputation of missing data. Multiple imputation of missing data minimizes loss of subjects who have missing data and thus preserves power to detect hypothesized effects. Multiple imputation was conducted in SAS in three steps. First, 20 data sets were imputed from the available data, with missing data on predeployment variables imputed from other predeployment variables and missing data on postdeployment variables imputed from other postdeployment variables. Second, in each of the 20 data sets, differences between the OSCAR-trained and control groups on the postdeployment outcomes were estimated using weighted, cluster-adjusted logistic regression models. Third, the parameter estimates representing differences between the OSCAR-trained and control groups on the postdeployment outcomes were aggregated across the 20 imputed datasets to generate a single set of parameter estimates.

In addition to examining OSCAR's effects on key outcomes, we examined variation in outcomes by battalion among only the OSCAR-trained battalions. This analysis was intended to illuminate possible variation in the implementation of OSCAR across battalions. Although such variation, if identified, could plausibly be attributed to many sources other than variation in the implementation of OSCAR, evidence of variation in outcomes by battalion would be consistent with the notion of cross-battalion variation in the implementation of OSCAR. Like we did in our analytical approach to estimating OSCAR's effects on outcomes, we estimated a series of multivariate regression models in which each outcome was regressed on a set of predictors that included the battalion modeled as a fixed effect represented by a set of dummy-coded indicators, with the battalion that was known to have received OSCAR training with high fidelity to the training guidelines serving as the reference group. Other baseline characteristics and deployment experiences were controlled for in all models.

Supplemental Descriptive Statistics from the Individual Marine Survey

This appendix contains additional descriptive statistics on the Marines who participated in the individual Marine survey component of the OSCAR evaluation. Specifically, we present comparisons between the entire sample of Marines and the broader population of active-duty and reservist Marines of rank O6 or lower who deployed to Iraq or Afghanistan in 2010 or 2011 on sociodemographic and service history characteristics (Table D.1). We also present comparisons between Marines in the OSCAR-trained and control battalions on T1 characteristics and deployment experiences (Table D.2) and T2 outcomes (Table D.3). The tests of statistical significance of differences between Marines in OSCAR-trained and control battalions reported in Tables D.2 and D.3 adjusted for clustering of Marines within battalions but did not make any other statistical adjustments (i.e., imputation of missing data, controlling for other variables, or propensity score weighting).

Sociodemographic and Service History Characteristics of the Final Sample of Marines Compared with the Broader Population of Marines

To determine how closely our sample resembled the larger population of active-duty and reservist Marines who deployed to Iraq or Afghanistan during the same period as the Marines who participated in this survey, we obtained administrative data from the Defense Manpower Data Center on the entire population of Marines of ranks E1–E9 and O1–O6 who deployed to Iraq or Afghanistan during 2010 or 2011 and compared their sociodemographic and service history characteristics with those of our sample. As shown in Table D.1, the sample of Marines in the current study differed from the broader population of Marines on several characteristics. Relative to the broader population, the current sample contains higher proportions of Marines who are under the age of 25, are junior enlisted, are unmarried, do not have children, and reported a history of one or more deployments to Iraq or Afghanistan prior to enrollment in this study.

Table D.1
Sociodemographic and Service History Characteristics of Individual Marine Survey Participants and
All Marines of Rank O6 or Lower Who Deployed to Iraq or Afghanistan in 2010 or 2011

| Characteristic | Individual Marine Survey Participants (N = 1,307) | | All Marines of Rank O6 or Lower Who Deployed to Iraq or Afghanistan in 2010 or 2011 (N = 32,854) |
	Percentage	95% CI	Percentage
Rank*			
E1–E3*	70	60.5–79.4	38
E4–E9*	26	18.3–33.8	49
Officer*	4	1.9–6.0	11
Under 25 years old*	78	71.7–84.6	61
Race or ethnicity			
White	70	65.5–75.4	72
Black	7	3.7–10.2	8
Hispanic*	19	15.3–22.0	13
Other	4	2.8–5.2	3
Married*	30	23.3–36.5	48
Has one child or more*	20	16.6–23.0	28
One or more previous deployments to Iraq or Afghanistan since 2001	34	25.0–43.2	25

* The population value for all Marines falls outside the 95-percent CI around the corresponding point estimate
for the sample of individual Marine survey participants, suggesting that the population value differs significantly
from the point estimate for the sample of survey participants.

Table D.2
Descriptive Statistics of Marines in the Final Sample and in OSCAR-Trained and Control Battalions on Characteristics and Deployment Experiences

Characteristic	Entire Sample (*N* = 1,307)	Control (*n* = 468)	OSCAR-Trained (*n* = 839)
Covariates and Levels of Outcomes Assessed in the T1 Survey			
		Percentage	
Rank†			
E1–E3	70	58	77
E4–E9	26	36	20
Officer	4	6	3
Age 25 or older*	22	30	17
Race or ethnicity			
White	70	68	72
Black	7	10	5
Hispanic	19	18	19
Other	4	4	4
Married	30	33	29
Has one child or more†	20	23	18
History of at least one deployment at baseline	34	28	37
Infantry (versus service-support) battalion[a]	57	0	89
Number of stress classes attended at baseline			
0	12	4	17
1–3	39	36	41
4 or more	49	61	43
Lifetime history of potentially traumatic events			
Natural disaster, fire or explosion, motor vehicle accident, other accident, or exposure to toxic substance	77	78	76
Physical assault, assault with weapon, combat, or captivity	55	50	58
Sexual assault or other unwanted sexual experience*	6	8	5
Witnessed violent death or experienced sudden, unexpected death of loved one*	50	46	52
Life-threatening illness or injury	13	13	12
Caused serious injury or death of another*	17	10	21
Experienced other very stressful event	40	37	41

Table D.2—Continued

Characteristic	Entire Sample (N = 1,307)	Control (n = 468)	OSCAR-Trained (n = 839)
Use of social resources for help with stress problems			
Fellow Marine	75	77	74
Leader*	50	56	46
Chaplain	20	25	17
Corpsman*	23	18	26
Unit medical officer	11	11	12
Any*[b]	82	86	80
Recommended resources to peer for help with stress problems			
Fellow Marine	85	87	84
Leader*	67	73	64
Chaplain*	56	66	51
Corpsman	38	31	42
Unit medical officer	26	28	25
Any*[b]	90	93	89
Current zone of the Combat and Operational Stress Continuum			
Green	45	44	46
Yellow	42	44	41
Orange or red	13	13	14
Current high-risk alcohol use	33	36	32
	M (SE)		
Expectancies regarding stress response and recovery[c]	4.0 (0.0)	4.0 (0.0)	4.0 (0.0)
Perceived support for help-seeking[d]	3.1 (0.0)	3.2 (0.0)	3.1 (0.0)
Unit support[e]	3.4 (0.0)	3.3 (0.0)	3.4 (0.0)
Lifetime history of PTSD symptom severity[f]	33.6 (0.4)	33.4 (0.9)	33.7 (0.6)
Past-month depressive symptoms[g]	1.1 (0.1)	1.1 (0.1)	1.2 (0.1)
General health[h]	71.3 (1.2)	72.4 (1.3)	70.7 (1.9)
Occupational impairment[i]	1.8 (0.0)	1.8 (0.1)	1.7 (0.1)
Deployment Experiences Assessed in T2 Survey			
	M(SE)		
Combat experiences during deployment[†j]	10.9 (0.9)	9.4 (0.5)	11.8 (1.3)
Peritraumatic distress[k]	22.1 (0.5)	21.5 (0.4)	22.5 (0.7)
Deployment environment*[l]	59.1 (2.0)	54.1 (0.9)	62.0 (1.8)

Table D.2—Continued

Characteristic	Entire Sample (*N* = 1,307)	Control (*n* = 468)	OSCAR-Trained (*n* = 839)

NOTE: All estimates and tests of significance referenced above adjust for clustering of Marines within battalions. Wald chi-squared tests of significance were conducted to compare the Marines in OSCAR-trained and control battalions on all of the variables in the table.

* Statistically significant differences between OSCAR-trained and control battalions at $p < 0.05$.

† Statistical comparison with a p-value less than 0.10 but greater than 0.05.

[a] The significance test to compare the proportions of Marines in OSCAR-trained and control battalions who were sampled from infantry versus service-support battalions could not be computed because there were no infantry battalions in the control group.

[b] *Any* resource used or recommended to a fellow Marine for help with stress problems refers to having used or recommended one or more of the five resources: fellow Marine, leader, chaplain, corpsman, or unit medical officer.

[c] Expectancies regarding stress response and recovery were measured on a scale on which possible scores range from 1 to 5, where higher scores indicate more-positive, healthier expectancies regarding stress response and recovery.

[d] Perceived support for help-seeking was measured on a scale on which possible scores range from 1 to 5, where higher scores indicate greater perceived support for help-seeking.

[e] Unit support was measured on a scale on which possible scores range from 1 to 5, where higher scores indicate more-positive perceptions of unit support.

[f] Lifetime history of PTSD symptom severity was measured with a modified version of the PCL-C on which possible scores range from 17 to 85, where higher scores indicate greater severity of PTSD symptoms experienced in one's lifetime.

[g] Past-month depressive symptoms were measured with the PHQ-2. The two items on this scale were summed to obtain a composite scale score on which possible scores range from 0 to 6, where higher scores indicate more-frequent depressive symptoms experienced in the past month.

[h] General health was measured with a single item from the SF-12. Possible scores range from 0 to 100, with higher scores indicating more-positive self-perceptions of overall health.

[i] Occupational impairment was measured on a scale on which possible scores range from 1 to 5, where higher scores indicate greater occupational impairment.

[j] Combat experiences during deployment were assessed on a scale that ranges from 0 to 40, where higher scores indicate more-frequent exposure to more types of combat experiences.

[k] Peritraumatic distress was measured on a scale on which possible scores range from 15 to 75, where higher scores indicate more-severe peritraumatic distress experienced during the most stressful event that occurred during the respondent's most recent deployment.

[l] Deployment environment was measured on a scale on which possible scores range from 20 to 100, where higher scores indicate greater levels of irritation and discomfort experienced during the respondent's most recent deployment.

Table D.3
Descriptive Statistics of Marines in the Final Sample and in OSCAR-Trained and Control Battalions on T2 Outcomes

Characteristic	Entire Sample (*N* = 1,307)	Control (*n* = 468)	OSCAR-Trained (*n* = 839)
	Percentage		
Use of social resources for help with stress problems			
Fellow Marine†	69	65	72
Leader	42	42	42
Chaplain	20	26	17
Corpsman	27	20	31
Unit medical officer*	11	14	10
Any	77	76	78
Recommended resources to peer for help with stress problems			
Fellow Marine	83	79	86
Leader	61	60	61
Chaplain	56	63	53
Corpsman†	48	38	53
Unit medical officer	29	32	28
Any[a]	89	88	89
Current zone of the Combat and Operational Stress Continuum			
Green	41	43	40
Yellow	42	40	43
Orange or red	17	17	16
Current probable PTSD	23	18	25
Current probable MDD	22	19	24
Current high-risk alcohol use	26	23	28
	M (SE)		
Expectancies about stress response and recovery[b]	4.0 (0.0)	4.0 (0.0)	4.0 (0.1)
Perceived support for help-seeking[c]	3.1 (0.1)	3.0 (0.0)	3.1 (0.1)
Unit support[d]	3.2 (0.1)	3.1 (0.0)	3.2 (0.1)
General health[e]	64.8 (2.2)	64.5 (1.5)	64.9 (3.4)
Occupational impairment[f]	1.9 (0.1)	1.9 (0.0)	1.9 (0.1)

Table D.3—Continued

Characteristic	Entire Sample (N = 1,307)	Control (n = 468)	OSCAR-Trained (n = 839)

NOTE: All estimates and tests of significance referenced above adjust for clustering of Marines within battalions. Wald chi-squared tests of significance were conducted to compare the Marines in OSCAR-trained and control battalions on all of the variables in the table.

* Statistically significant differences between OSCAR-trained and control battalions at $p < 0.05$.

† Statistical comparison with a p-value less than 0.10 but greater than 0.05.

[a] *Any* resource used or recommended to a fellow Marine for help with stress problems refers to having used or recommended one or more of the five resources: fellow Marine, leader, chaplain, corpsman, or unit medical officer.

[b] Expectancies regarding stress response and recovery were measured on a scale on which possible scores range from 1 to 5, where higher scores indicate more-positive, healthier expectancies regarding stress response and recovery.

[c] Perceived support for help-seeking was measured on a scale on which possible scores range from 1 to 5, where higher scores indicate greater perceived support for help-seeking.

[d] Unit support was measured on a scale on which possible scores range from 1 to 5, where higher scores indicate more-positive perceptions of unit support.

[e] General health was measured with a single item from the SF-12. Possible scores range from 0 to 100, with higher scores indicating more-positive self-perceptions of overall health.

[f] Occupational impairment was measured on a scale on which possible scores range from 1 to 5, where higher scores indicate greater occupational impairment.

Sensitivity Analyses for the Individual Marine Survey

This appendix contains detailed results from two sets of sensitivity analyses of the treatment effect estimates (i.e., effect of having been in an OSCAR-trained versus non–OSCAR-trained battalion on outcomes): (1) multivariate models estimated with multiple imputation of missing data to assess the extent of sample bias that might have resulted from listwise deletion of cases in multivariate models that were not adjusted for missing data (Table E.1) and (2) multivariate models estimated within the subset of service-support (noninfantry) battalions in an attempt to disentangle OSCAR's effects from that of battalion type on outcomes (Table E.2). All multivariate models were estimated with adjustment for clustering of participants within battalions and T1 characteristics and deployment experiences. For both sets of analyses, the treatment effect estimates are juxtaposed with treatment effect estimates obtained on the full sample without adjustment for missing data, which were presented in Chapter Three.

Multiple Imputation of Missing Data

As shown in Table E.1, for every outcome, the statistical significance of the treatment effect estimate at $p < 0.05$ (i.e., whether the estimate was statistically significant or not) was the same in multivariate models estimated with and without multiple imputation of missing data. In addition, the magnitude of effect (size of the odds ratio [OR]) was very similar in both models for every outcome. Thus, it appears that there was minimal sample bias from the exclusion of cases with missing data on one or more variables (i.e., listwise deletion) in the multivariate models estimated without imputation of missing data.

Disentangling OSCAR's Effects from Battalion Type

Because the receipt of OSCAR training was highly confounded with the type of battalion (infantry versus service support), we conducted a sensitivity analysis to disentangle OSCAR's effects training from those of battalion type. Specifically, for the six help-seeking outcomes on which OSCAR had significant effects in the full sample, we estimated OSCAR's effects within one type of battalion, the service-support battalions. By holding battalion type constant, we were able to isolate OSCAR's effects from those of battalion type. Thus, replication of the pattern of findings within one type of battalion would strengthen confidence that the effects observed in the full sample are attributable to OSCAR rather than battalion type. Because all infantry battalions had received OSCAR training, we were unable to examine

Table E.1
Comparison of Treatment Effect Estimates from Multivariate Models Estimated With and Without Multiple Imputation of Missing Data

Characteristic	Treatment Effect Estimates from Unadjusted Models (N = 972)		Treatment Effect Estimates from Models in Which Missing Data Were Imputed (N = 1,307)	
	OR	95% CI	OR	95% CI
Expectancies regarding stress response and recovery	0.96	0.60–1.54	1.10	0.66–1.82
Perceived support for help-seeking	1.12	0.69–1.80	1.35	0.80–2.28
Unit support	1.28	0.75–2.21	1.36	0.78–2.37
Use of social resources for help with stress problems				
Fellow Marine*	1.65	1.32–2.07	1.66	1.34–2.06
Leader*	1.37	1.10–1.72	1.38	1.03–1.85
Chaplain	0.80	0.64–1.01	0.87	0.62–1.22
Corpsman*	1.62	1.05–2.49	1.82	1.37–2.42
Unit medical officer	0.80	0.49–1.30	0.81	0.57–1.14
Any*	1.60	1.19–2.14	1.61	1.17–2.22
Recommended resources to peer for help with stress problems				
Fellow Marine*	1.83	1.45–2.31	1.74	1.35–2.24
Leader*	1.79	1.37–2.33	1.67	1.28–2.19
Chaplain	0.84	0.69–1.04	0.93	0.68–1.28
Corpsman*	2.00	1.44–2.78	2.07	1.55–2.76
Unit medical officer	0.92	0.55–1.55	0.97	0.69–1.36
Any*	1.64	1.26–2.15	1.59	1.18–2.15
Yellow, orange, or red stress zone	1.04	0.71–1.52	1.02	0.67–1.56
Current probable PTSD	1.38	0.91–2.09	1.20	0.76–1.90
Current probable MDD	1.52	0.93–2.49	1.28	0.82–2.01
Current high-risk alcohol use	1.04	0.66–1.62	1.12	0.72–1.73
General health	1.37	0.74–2.52	1.32	0.68–2.58
Occupational impairment	0.86	0.59–1.24	0.98	0.68–1.40

* The treatment effect on the outcome was statistically significant at $p < 0.05$.

[a] The sample size for each multivariate model ranged from 972 to 1,063 across the outcomes listed in the table.

Table E.2
Comparison of Multivariate Models Estimated in the Full Sample and in Service-Support Battalions

Characteristic	Treatment Effect Estimates in the Full Sample (N = 972)[a]		Treatment Effect Estimates in Service-Support Battalions Only (N = 416)[b]	
	OR	95% CI	OR	OR (95% CI LL, 95% CI UI)
Use of social resources for help with stress problems				
Fellow Marine	1.65*	1.32–2.07	2.05*	1.31–3.21
Leader	1.37*	1.10–1.72	1.30	0.57–2.96
Chaplain	0.80	0.64–1.01	0.41	0.16–1.07
Corpsman	1.62*	1.05–2.49	2.19	0.91–5.28
Unit medical officer	0.80	0.49–1.30	1.09	0.46–2.60
Any	1.60*	1.19–2.14	1.21	0.76–1.93
Recommended resources to peer for help with stress problems				
Fellow Marine	1.83*	1.45–2.31	2.57*	1.67–3.95
Leader	1.79*	1.37–2.33	1.54	0.87–2.75
Chaplain	0.84	0.69–1.04	0.77	0.43–1.38
Corpsman	2.00*	1.44–2.78	1.51*	1.04–2.21
Unit medical officer	0.92	0.55–1.55	1.02	0.41–2.52
Any	1.64*	1.26–2.15	3.31*	1.91–5.76

* The treatment effect on the outcome was statistically significant at $p < 0.05$.

[a] Treatment effect estimates on the full sample are from multivariate models with no adjustments for missing data. The sample size for each multivariate model ranged from 972 to 1,043 across the outcomes listed in the table.

[b] Treatment effect estimates on the subset of service-support battalions are from multivariate models with no adjustments for missing data. The total sample size for Marines in service-support battalions was 558, but with listwise deletion in multivariate models because of missing data on one or more variables, the sample size for each multivariate model ranged from 416 to 448 across the outcomes listed in the table.

OSCAR's effects (compared with the control group) within the infantry battalions. However, both OSCAR-trained and non–OSCAR-trained battalions were represented among the service-support battalions.

Within the subset of service-support battalions, we ran a series of multivariate models to estimate OSCAR's effects and determine whether the significant effects of OSCAR observed in the full sample would be replicated among this subset. The sample size of Marines in service-support battalions was less than half of the full sample size, which reduced power to detect significant effects of OSCAR in the smaller group. Accordingly, we anticipated that the significant effects of OSCAR observed in the full sample would be less likely to be significant in the smaller sample. Thus, we focused instead on comparing the full sample and subset of Marines in service-support battalions on the magnitude and direction of treatment effect estimates.

In the full sample (as described in Chapter Three), we found that OSCAR significantly increased the use of fellow Marines, leaders, corpsmen, and any one of the resources assessed for help with one's own stress problems, as well as having recommended fellow Marines, leaders, corpsmen, or any of these resources to peers for help with his or her stress problems. Not surprisingly, for four of these six outcomes, OSCAR's effects failed to attain statistical significance in the subset of Marines in service-support battalions. For the remaining two outcomes, however, OSCAR did have a significant effect among the Marines in service-support battalions. For every outcome, the direction of the effect was the same in the full sample and subset of Marines in service-support battalions (i.e., OSCAR increased these behaviors in both groups). The magnitude of effects was generally comparable across the two groups, except that the odds ratio for recommending the use of any resource to a peer was roughly twice as high among the service-support battalions as in the full sample. Given the replication of the general pattern of results obtained in the full sample among the Marines in service-support battalions, then, the significant effects of OSCAR on help-seeking behavior appear to be better attributable to OSCAR than to battalion type. Odds ratios and CIs for OSCAR's effects on the six outcomes that OSCAR significantly affected in the full sample are displayed in Table E.2 for both the full sample and the subset of Marines in service-support battalions.

APPENDIX F
Attrition Analysis for OSCAR Team Member Survey

Similar to the individual Marine survey, anecdotal reports from our POCs in the units surveyed indicate that the primary causes of attrition, i.e., loss of study participants between the T1 and T2 surveys, include transitions that often occur soon after redeployment, such as PCS or EAS. Marines who had PCS'ed or EAS'ed soon after redeployment were not available on base to complete the T2 survey when it was administered to their units.

To assess the extent to which the sample might have been biased by attrition between T1 and T2, we ran a series of cluster-adjusted bivariate binary logistic regressions predicting the odds of completing the T2 survey (versus not completing the T2 survey) from each of the items assessed in the T1 survey (see Table 4.1 in Chapter Four). The only T1 variables that significantly predicted the odds of T2 survey completion were frequency of depression consults (OR = 0.81, 95-percent CI [0.72–0.91]), perceived ease of providers talking to line leaders about the needs of Marines (OR = 0.83, 95-percent CI [0.70–0.99]), and expectations regarding OSCAR's impact on leaders' ability to access the appropriate level of care for Marines with stress problems (OR = 1.42, 95-percent CI [1.11–1.82]). Thus, participants who reported receiving less frequent consults for problems with depression, less positive perceptions of the ease with which providers could talk to line leaders about the needs of Marines, and more-positive expectations regarding OSCAR's impact on leaders' ability to access the appropriate level of care for Marines with stress problems had significantly greater odds of completing the T2 survey.

References

Assistant Secretary of Defense for Health Affairs, *Combat Stress Control (CSC) Programs*, Department of Defense Directive 6490.5, February 23, 1999; reissued as Department of Defense Instruction 6490.05 November 22, 2011. As of December 2, 2013:
http://biotech.law.lsu.edu/blaw/dodd/corres/pdf/d64905_022399/d64905p.pdf

Bartone, Paul T., "Resilience Under Military Operational Stress: Can Leaders Influence Hardiness?," *Military Psychology*, Vol. 18, Suppl., 2006, pp. S131–S148.

Bellg, Albert J., Belinda Borrelli, Barbara Resnick, Jacki Hecht, Daryl Sharp Minicucci, Marcia Ory, Gbenga Ogedegbe, Denise Orwig, Denise Ernst, and Susan Czajkowski, "Enhancing Treatment Fidelity in Health Behavior Change Studies: Best Practices and Recommendations from the NIH Behavior Change Consortium," *Health Psychology*, Vol. 23, No. 5, 2004, pp. 443–451.

Brewin, Chris R., "Systematic Review of Screening Instruments for Adults at Risk of PTSD," *Journal of Traumatic Stress*, Vol. 18, No. 1, 2005, pp. 53–62.

Brewin, Chris R., Bernice Andrews, and John D. Valentine, "Meta-Analysis of Risk Factors for Posttraumatic Stress Disorder in Trauma-Exposed Adults," *Journal of Consulting and Clinical Psychology*, Vol. 68, No. 5, 2000, pp. 748–766.

Brymer, Melissa, Christopher Layne, Anne Jacobs, Robert Pynoos, Josef Ruzek, Alan Steinberg, Eric Vernberg, and Patricia Watson, "Psychological First Aid Field Operations Guide," 2006. As of December 2, 2013:
http://www.nctsn.org/sites/default/files/pfa/english/1-psyfirstaid_final_complete_manual.pdf

Bush, K., D. R. Kivlahan, M. B. McDonell, S. D. Fihn, and K. A. Bradley, "The Audit Alcohol Consumption Questions (AUDIT-C): An Effective Brief Screening Test for Problem Drinking—Ambulatory Care Quality Improvement Project (ACQUIP): Alcohol Use Disorders Identification Test," *Archives of Internal Medicine*, Vol. 158, No. 16, 1998, pp. 1789–1795.

Chief of Naval Operations and Commandant of the Marine Corps, *Combat and Operational Stress Control*, Marine Corps Reference Publication 6-11C and Navy Tactics, Techniques, and Procedures 1-15M, December 20, 2010. As of December 2, 2013:
http://www.uscg.mil/worklife/docs/pdf/Navy_and_Marine_Corps_OSC_Doctrine_Dec_2010%5b1%5d.pdf

Dawson, Deborah A., Bridget F. Grant, Frederick S. Stinson, and Yuan Zhou, "Effectiveness of the Derived Alcohol Use Disorders Identification Test (AUDIT-C) in Screening for Alcohol Use Disorders and Risk Drinking in the US General Population," *Alcoholism: Clinical and Experimental Research*, Vol. 29, No. 5, 2005, pp. 844–854.

Department of Veterans Affairs and Department of Defense, "VA/DoD Clinical Practice Guideline for Substance Abuse Disorders, Version 2.0," 2009.

Dickstein, Benjamin D., Carmen P. McLean, Jim Mintz, Lauren M. Conoscenti, Maria M. Steenkamp, Trisha A. Benson, William C. Isler, Alan L. Peterson, and Brett T. Litz, "Unit Cohesion and PTSD Symptom Severity in Air Force Medical Personnel," *Military Medicine*, Vol. 175, No. 7, 2010, pp. 482–486.

Farmer, Carrie M., Christine Anne Vaughan, Jeffrey Garnett, and Robin M. Weinick, *Pre-Deployment Stress, Mental Health, and Help-Seeking Behaviors Among Marines*, Santa Monica, Calif.: RAND Corporation, RR-218-OSD, 2014. As of March 11, 2015:
http://www.rand.org/pubs/research_reports/RR218.html

Graubard, Barry I., and Edward L. Korn, "Predictive Margins with Survey Data," *Biometrics*, Vol. 55, No. 2, 1999, pp. 652–659.

Gray, Matt J., Brett T. Litz, Julie L. Hsu, and Thomas W. Lombardo, "Psychometric Properties of the Life Events Checklist," *Assessment*, Vol. 11, No. 4, December 1, 2004, pp. 330–341.

Hays, Ron D., Cathy Donald Sherbourne, and Rebecca M. Mazel, "The RAND 36-Item Health Survey 1.0," *Health Economics*, Vol. 2, No. 3, 1993, pp. 217–227.

Headquarters Department of the Army, *Combat and Operational Stress Control*, Field Manual 4-02.51, July 2006. As of March 5, 2014:
http://armypubs.army.mil/doctrine/DR_pubs/dr_a/pdf/fm4_02x51.pdf

Hoge, Charles W., Carl A. Castro, Stephen C. Messer, Dennis McGurk, Dave I. Cotting, and Robert L. Koffman, "Combat Duty in Iraq and Afghanistan, Mental Health Problems, and Barriers to Care," *New England Journal of Medicine*, Vol. 351, No. 1, 2004, pp. 13–22.

Institute of Medicine, Committee on the Assessment of Ongoing Efforts in the Treatment of Posttraumatic Stress Disorder, Board on the Health of Select Populations, *Treatment for Posttraumatic Stress Disorder in Military and Veteran Populations: Final Assessment*, Washington, D.C., June 20, 2014. As of March 11, 2015:
http://www.iom.edu/Reports/2014/
Treatment-for-Posttraumatic-Stress-Disorder-in-Military-and-Veteran-Populations-Final-Assessment.aspx

Kessler, Ronald C., Catherine Barber, Arne Beck, Patricia Berglund, Paul D. Cleary, David McKenas, Nico Pronk, Gregory Simon, and Paul Stang, "The World Health Organization Health and Work Performance Questionnaire (HPQ)," *Journal of Occupational and Environmental Medicine*, Vol. 45, No. 2, 2003, pp. 156–174.

Kim, Paul, Jeffrey Thomas, Joshua Wilk, Carl Castro, and Charles Hoge, "Stigma, Barriers to Care, and Use of Mental Health Services Among Active Duty and National Guard Soldiers After Combat," *Psychiatric Services*, Vol. 61, No. 6, 2010, pp. 582–588.

King, Lynda A., Daniel W. King, Dawne S. Vogt, Jeffrey Knight, and Rita E. Samper, "Deployment Risk and Resilience Inventory: A Collection of Measures for Studying Deployment-Related Experiences of Military Personnel and Veterans," *Military Psychology*, Vol. 18, No. 2, 2006, pp. 89–120.

Kroenke, Kurt, Robert L. Spitzer, and Janet B. W. Williams, "The PHQ-9: Validity of a Brief Depression Severity Measure," *Journal of General Internal Medicine*, Vol. 16, No. 9, 2001, pp. 606–613.

———, "The Patient Health Questionnaire–2: Validity of a Two-Item Depression Screener," *Medical Care*, Vol. 41, No. 11, 2003, pp. 1284–1292.

Kroenke, Kurt, Tara W. Strine, Robert L. Spitzer, Janet B. W. Williams, Joyce T. Berry, and Ali H. Mokdad, "The PHQ-8 as a Measure of Current Depression in the General Population," *Journal of Affective Disorders*, Vol. 114, No. 1–3, 2009, pp. 163–173.

Löwe, Bernd, Kurt Kroenke, Wolfgang Herzog, and Kerstin Gräfe, "Measuring Depression Outcome with a Brief Self-Report Instrument: Sensitivity to Change of the Patient Health Questionnaire (PHQ-9)," *Journal of Affective Disorders*, Vol. 81, No. 1, 2004, pp. 61–66.

Mansfield, Alyssa J., Jason Williams, Laurel L. Hourani, and Lorraine A. Babeu, "Measurement Invariance of Posttraumatic Stress Disorder Symptoms Among U.S. Military Personnel," *Journal of Traumatic Stress*, Vol. 23, No. 1, 2010, pp. 91–99.

Meredith, Lisa S., Cathy D. Sherbourne, Sarah J. Gaillot, Lydia Hansell, Hans V. Ritschard, Andrew M. Parker, and Glenda Wrenn, *Promoting Psychological Resilience in the U.S. Military*, Santa Monica, Calif.: RAND Corporation, MG-996-OSD, 2011. As of November 3, 2013:
http://www.rand.org/pubs/monographs/MG996

Nash, William P., "Operational Stress Control and Readiness (OSCAR): The United States Marine Corps Initiative to Deliver Mental Health Services to Operating Forces," in North Atlantic Treaty Organization Science and Technology Organization, *Human Dimensions in Military Operations—Military Leaders' Strategies for Addressing Stress and Psychological Support, Meeting Proceedings*, Neuilly-sur-Seine, France: North Atlantic Treaty Organisation Research and Technology Organisation, RTO-MP-HFM-134, Paper 25, 2006, pp. 25-1– 25-10. As of March 12, 2015:
http://ftp.rta.nato.int/public//PubFullText/RTO/MP/RTO-MP-HFM-134///MP-HFM-134-25.pdf

———, "US Marine Corps and Navy Combat and Operational Stress Continuum Model: A Tool for Leaders," in Elspeth Cameron Ritchie, ed., *Combat and Operational Behavioral Health: Textbook of Military Psychiatry*, Washington, D.C.: Office of the Surgeon General and Borden Institute, 2011. As of December 2, 2013:
https://ke.army.mil/bordeninstitute/published_volumes/combat_operational/CBM-ch7-final.pdf

Nash, William P., G. Goldwasser, J. B. Lohr, D. G. Baker, S.E. Nunnink, and D. Siegmann, "Poster Session— The Peritraumatic Behavior Questionnaire: A Proposed Observer-Rated Measure of Combat-Related Stress for Utilization in the War Zone," *Veterans Affairs Mental Health Summit*, Baltimore, Md., 2009.

Nash, William P., Lillian Krantz, Nathan Stein, Richard J. Westphal, and Brett Litz, "Comprehensive Soldier Fitness, Battlemind, and the Stress Continuum Model: Military Organizational Approaches to Prevention," in Josef I. Ruzek, Paula P. Schnurr, Jennifer J. Vasterling, and Matthew J. Friedman, eds., *Caring for Veterans with Deployment-Related Stress Disorders: Iraq, Afghanistan, and Beyond*, Washington, D.C.: American Psychological Association, 2011.

Nash, William P., and Patricia J. Watson, "Review of VA/DoD Clinical Practice Guideline on Management of Acute Stress and Interventions to Prevent Posttraumatic Stress Disorder," *Journal of Rehabilitation Research and Development*, Vol. 49, No. 6, 2012, pp. 637–648.

Nash, William P., Richard J. Westphal, Patricia J. Watson, and Brett T. Litz, "Combat and Operational Stress First Aid: Caregiver Training Manual," 2010. As of December 2, 2013:
http://www.alsbom-gm.org/files/COSFA%20NAVY%20TM.pdf

Naval Center for Combat and Operational Stress Control, "5 Core Leadership Functions," NCCOSC, undated. As of September 17, 2012:
http://www.med.navy.mil/sites/nmcsd/nccosc/leadersV2/infoAndTools/5CoreLeadershipFunctions/Pages/default.aspx

Office of the Inspector General, *Evaluation Report on the Management of Combat Stress Control in the Department of Defense*, Arlington, Va.: U.S. Department of Defense, Report 96-079, February 29, 1996. As of December 2, 2013:
http://www.dodig.mil/audit/reports/fy96/96-079.pdf

Ozer, Emily J., Suzanne R. Best, Tami L. Lipsey, and Daniel S. Weiss, "Predictors of Posttraumatic Stress Disorder and Symptoms in Adults: A Meta-Analysis," *Psychological Bulletin*, Vol. 129, No. 1, 2003, pp. 52–73.

Pornpitakpan, Chanthika, "The Persuasiveness of Source Credibility: A Critical Review of Five Decades' Evidence," *Journal of Applied Social Psychology*, Vol. 34, No. 2, 2004, pp. 243–281.

Ruggiero, Kenneth J., Kevin Del Ben, Joseph R. Scotti, and Aline E. Rabalais, "Psychometric Properties of the PTSD Checklist—Civilian Version," *Journal of Traumatic Stress*, Vol. 16, No. 5, 2003, pp. 495–502.

Ryan, Gery W., Carrie M. Farmer, David M. Adamson, and Robin M. Weinick, *A Program Manager's Guide for Program Improvement in Ongoing Psychological Health and Traumatic Brain Injury Programs: The RAND Toolkit*, Volume 4, Santa Monica, Calif.: RAND Corporation, RR-487/4-OSD, 2014. As of January 23, 2014:
http://www.rand.org/pubs/research_reports/RR487z4

Saks, Alan M., and Monica Belcourt, "An Investigation of Training Activities and Transfer of Training in Organizations," *Human Resource Management*, Vol. 45, No. 4, 2006, pp. 629–648.

Schafer, Joseph L., and John W. Graham, "Missing Data: Our View of the State of the Art," *Psychological Methods*, Vol. 7, No. 2, 2002, pp. 147–177.

Schell, Terry L., and Grant N. Marshall, "Survey of Individuals Previously Deployed for OEF/OIF," in Terri L. Tanielian, Lisa H. Jaycox, Terry L. Schell, Grant N. Marshall, M. Audrey Burnam, Christine Eibner, Benjamin R. Karney, Lisa S. Meredith, Jeanne S. Ringel, and Mary E. Vaiana, eds., *Invisible Wounds of War: Summary and Recommendations for Addressing Psychological and Cognitive Injuries*, Santa Monica, Calif.: RAND Corporation, MG-720/1-CCF, 2008. As of September 10, 2013:
http://www.rand.org/pubs/monographs/MG720z1

Setodji, Claude Messan, Maren Scheuner, James S. Pankow, Roger S. Blumenthal, Haiying Chen, and Emmett Keeler, "A Graphical Method for Assessing Risk Factor Threshold Values Using the Generalized Additive Model: The Multi-Ethnic Study of Atherosclerosis," *Health Services and Outcomes Research Methodology*, Vol. 12, No. 1, March 1, 2012, pp. 62–79.

Shepard, Ben, *A War of Nerves: Soldiers and Psychiatrists in the Twentieth Century*, Cambridge, Mass.: Harvard University Press, 2001.

Shils, Edward A., and Morris Janowitz, "Cohesion and Disintegration in the Wehrmacht in World War II," *Public Opinion Quarterly*, Vol. 12, No. 2, June 20, 1948, pp. 280–315.

U.S. Marine Corps, *Operational Stress Control and Readiness Training Guidance*, Marine Administrative Message 597/11, October 7, 2011. As of December 2, 2013:
http://www.marines.mil/News/Messages/MessagesDisplay/tabid/13286/Article/110997/operational-stress-control-and-readiness-training-guidance.aspx

———, *Never Leave a Marine Behind Annual Suicide Prevention Training and Master Training Team Requirements*, Marine Administrative Message 524/12, September 20, 2012. As of March 10, 2013:
http://www.marines.mil/News/Messages/MessagesDisplay/tabid/13286/Article/110342/never-leave-a-Marine-behind-annual-suicide-prevention-training-and-master-train.aspx

Vogt, Dawne S., Susan P. Proctor, Daniel W. King, Lynda A. King, and Jennifer J. Vasterling, "Validation of Scales from the Deployment Risk and Resilience Inventory in a Sample of Operation Iraqi Freedom Veterans," *Assessment*, Vol. 15, No. 4, 2008, pp. 391–403.

Ware, John E., Jr., Mark Kosinski, and Susan D. Keller, "A 12-Item Short-Form Health Survey: Construction of Scales and Preliminary Tests of Reliability and Validity," *Medical Care*, Vol. 34, No. 3, 1996, pp. 220–233.

Warner, Christopher H., George N. Appenzeller, Thomas Grieger, Slava Belenkiy, Jill Breitbach, Jessica Parker, Carolynn M. Warner, and Charles Hoge, "Importance of Anonymity to Encourage Honest Reporting in Mental Health Screening After Combat Deployment," *Archives of General Psychiatry*, Vol. 68, No. 10, 2011, pp. 1063–1071.

Weathers, Frank W., Jennifer A. Huska, and Terrence M. Keane, "PCL-C for DSM-IV," Boston, Mass.: National Center for PTSD-Behavioral Science Division, 1991.

Weathers, Frank, B. T. Litz, D. S. Herman, Jennifer A. Huska, and Terrence M. Keane, "The PTSD Checklist: Reliability, Validity, and Diagnostic Utility," paper presented at Annual Meeting of the International Society for Traumatic Stress Studies, San Antonio, Texas, 1993.

Weinick, Robin M., Ellen Burke Beckjord, Carrie M. Farmer, Laurie T. Martin, Emily M. Gillen, Joie Acosta, Michael P. Fisher, Jeffrey Garnett, Gabriella C. Gonzalez, Todd C. Helmus, Lisa H. Jaycox, Kerry Reynolds, Nicholas Salcedo, and Deborah M. Scharf, *Programs Addressing Psychological Health and Traumatic Brain Injury Among U.S. Military Servicemembers and Their Families*, Santa Monica, Calif.: RAND Corporation, TR-950-OSD, 2011. As of December 5, 2013:
http://www.rand.org/pubs/technical_reports/TR950

Wessely, Simon, "Victimhood and Resilience," *New England Journal of Medicine*, Vol. 353, No. 6, 2005, pp. 548–550.

———, "Twentieth-Century Theories on Combat Motivation and Breakdown," *Journal of Contemporary History*, Vol. 41, No. 2, 2006, pp. 268–286.

Wright, Kathleen M., Oscar A. Cabrera, Paul D. Bliese, Amy B. Adler, Charles W. Hoge, and Carl A. Castro, "Stigma and Barriers to Care in Soldiers Postcombat," *Psychological Services*, Vol. 6, No. 2, 2009, pp. 108–116.